# Celebration

Margaret Spufford is well known as an influential seventeenth-century historian and is also a Benedictine tertiary. An oblate of St Mary's Abbey, West Malling, she is also a Research Professor of Social and Local History at Roehampton Institute, London, a Doctor of Letters of Cambridge University, and a Fellow of the British Academy.

For Peter, who has lived with the raw material for over twenty-five years, and Richard, who first asked me to talk about pain, and has given so prodigally of his time to help form the results

# MARGARET SPUFFORD

# *Celebration*

COWLEY PUBLICATIONS
*Cambridge* ◆ *Boston*
*Massachusetts*

Published in the United States of America by Cowley
Publications, a division of the Society of St. John the
Evangelist. No portion of this book may be reproduced, stored
in or introduced into a retrieval system, or transmitted, in any
form or by any means—including photocopying—without the
prior written permission of Cowley Publications,
except in the case of brief quotations embodied in
critical articles and reviews.

Library of Congress Cataloging-in-Publication Data
may be obtained from the Library of Congress,
Washington, D. C.
or from Cowley Publications.

ISBN: 1-56101-129-0

Printed and bound in Great Britain by
Biddles Ltd, Guildford and King's Lynn

Cowley Publications
28 Temple Place
Boston, Massachusetts 02111

# Contents

# *Forewords*

What makes *Celebration* so remarkable and so authoritative is that it is a study of suffering from the inside. Dr Spufford writes from pain and in pain: from and in the physical pain of her own incurable disease – from and in the mental pain of her daughter's incurable disease. She writes not of pain recollected in tranquillity, but of pain as her present experience and her lifelong expectation. Yet she writes with the cool and clear objectivity of her calling as a professional historian and the theological insight of a Christian mind steeped in contemplation.

As I read *Celebration* I kept thinking of Bonhoeffer's *Letters and Papers from Prison*. To Dr Spufford's "captivity", as to Bonhoeffer's, no end is in view, no release to be expected: and she would certainly say, as he did, that "only a suffering God can help us". And for her, as for him, the reality and the presence of the suffering God is the source of a shining and almost palpable joy. And, again like Bonhoeffer, Dr Spufford gives us, almost as asides, many precise and crystal-clear comments on great matters of our day – in her case on such diverse matters as family life, medical ethics and intellectual creativity.

No theologian may now write about the problems of suffering without reference to this book. In the light of it no glib "answer" to the problem can be taken seriously: but anyone who is bewildered and morally affronted by his or her own pain will do well to follow Dr Spufford along the painful steps of her austere but joyful pilgrimage.

It would be an impertinence to praise this book: all we may do is thank Dr Spufford – and her family – for it.

W. H. VANSTONE

We read a lot about the triumphs of modern technological medicine but its practitioners are becoming increasingly concerned about the way in which such means are related to the ends that they are supposed to serve: what cart is the scientific horse supposed to be pulling and where is it going? Dr Spufford's book is about one such "triumph" and the effect it has had on her family's life. At one level as agreeable as possible, complete with personal and academic fulfilment – involving, as Freud put it, the two desiderata of love and work: and on the other difficult, even tragic, and unselfconsciously heroic. It is a book that all those who need reminding that medicine is an art that uses science, whether as givers or receivers, would gain a lot from reading – and reading reflectively despite the pain and doubt that it makes explicit. It raises much more important questions in relation to medical practice and ethics than we have got used to being asked by politicians, moral philosophers and patients preoccupied with its economics, sociology and accountability at a superficial level. One such question is Qui bono? Another, are the good intentions with which the road to hell is said to be paved those carried out or those not carried out? I suggest that all sixth formers hoping to embark on a medical career should read this book and every hospital Chaplain.

JOHN A. DAVIS
Professor of Paediatrics in
the University of Cambridge

# Acknowledgements

There are many people I would like to thank who have been helpful over twenty years. If any are omitted here, I would be grateful for their forgiveness.

There are my colleagues, Gillian Sutherland and Rosamond McKitterick, who have given me much support over the last few difficult years. The Principal of Newnham College, Miss Sheila Browne, was first, I think, to suggest I write a non-historical book.

I lacked parents, but instead I had my elder sister Jean and her husband Dick, and mother-in-law, Nancy, as well as Hugh and Geraldine Prew, and Herbert and Josceline Finberg.

There are friends, above all Ione Shaw and Jack Ravensdale, Colin and Myrna Richmond, Patricia Beattie, Anna Bidder, Susan Cattermole, and Susan Gomme, Virginia and George Holt, Donald Nicholl, Marjorie McIntosh, Mary Pratt, Charlotte and David Vincent, Pat White, Esther de Waal, and latterly, Martin and Teresa Brett, and Eamon Duffy. There are also those who came to help, or to be taught, and became friends, above all Kirsten Carlsen, Birgit Mielke, and Gertrud Messerschmidt. Among their number, too, were Louise Hodgson, Elizabeth Key, Sally Weightman, Susan Paine, Alison Tyler, Judith Maltby, Ken Parker, Eric Carlson, Ulrike Balser, Helen Robinshaw, Sarah and Geoff Schrecker, Pauline Möckel, Roger Smith, Mrs Jepson, Mary Darlington, Sandra Williamson, and Jane Baldwin. Sue Glennie ·typed this at high speed, and thereby made this work possible for me. Carolyn Busfield ran off the fluid charts in the History Department at Keele.

Amongst doctors, I am deeply indebted to Brian Davy. There are also the GPs who treated us as a family, and never merely as "cases" of osteoporosis and cystinosis, Ralph Canter, Pam Kenny and Ann Kemp. There are paediatricians who treated parents as people, above all Professor Otto Wolff, Professor John Davis, John Harries, and Susan Rigden. Latterly there have been other consultants, notably Paul Siklos, and Gwyn Williams. There have been paediatric nurses who loved Bridget, and made space for her mother and her mother's paperwork. The first of them was Sister Hensman. Sister Elizabeth Wilson trained me to put a gastric tube down, and thereby gave us our family unity back. The last of them was Sister Theo Mannie. Amongst schoolteachers, we owe a special debt to Miss Margaret Cooper and Mrs Duggan of Seabridge Primary School, Mr Hollinghurst of Blackfriars School, Newcastle-under-Lyme, and Mrs Fiona Unwin.

There have been priests who have helped, or listened. Among them are Metropolitan Anthony Bloom, Victor de Waal, Bishop Peter Walker, David Conner, Robert Mitchell, Harry Potter, and above all Richard Hunt. There have been other people who principally prayed, notably the Community of St Mary's Abbey, West Malling, and my oblate Mistress, Sister Elizabeth. I owe my acquaintance with Kathleen Raine to the Mother Abbess. To the Community above all I owe hospitality and support over many years, most recently while I have tried to write this book. My research students understood my going away to do so. They have also shown amazing patience with a supervisor whose teaching hours, and physical position, changed according to the degree of pain she was in, and how unwell her daughter was. Their generosity has enabled me to continue to teach. I would therefore also like to thank Amy Erickson, Chris Marsh, Derek Plumb, Bill Stevenson, Keith Stride, Matthew Storey, Moto Takahashi, Tessa Watt, and Helen Weinstein, for their care and forbearance.

In making any distinction of function between those who have ministered to me in different ways all this time, I make no distinction in importance. Those who have cleaned my floors and sorted the muddle around me, have been at least as vital to me as those who have measured the density of my bones, listened to me when I was in distress, looked after our daughter, or prayed for us. Some, at least, of these people have fulfilled more than one function. All categorization is misleading: yet a list in strict alphabetical order is perhaps even more misleading. I am very thankful to them all.

I knew I owed much to the novelist H.M. Prescott, but not how much, until I found I had used her words unconsciously under pressure at the end.

All my family urged me on. My son Francis read the typescript in his professional capacity, and has done some editorial work on it. My debt to my daughter Bridget is of course immeasurable. The invisible presence of my husband, Peter, stands behind every page.

Begun at St Mary's, West Malling
on the Feast of the Lady Julian, 1987.
Finished, Lent, 1988.

Mine eyes are ever looking unto the Lord:
for He shall pluck my feet out of the net.
Turn thou unto me, and have mercy upon me:
  for I am desolate and in misery.
The sorrows of my heart are enlarged:
  o bring thou me out of my troubles.
O keep my soul and deliver me: let me not be confounded,
  for I have put my trust in thee.
Let perfectness and righteous dealing wait upon me:
  for my hope hath been in thee.

Psalm 25


O God, you are my God, I seek you, my soul thirsts for you,
  my flesh faints for you as in a dry and weary land where no
  water is.
So I have looked upon you in the sanctuary, beholding your
  power and glory.
Because your steadfast love is better than life, my lips will
  praise you; so I will bless you as long as I live, I will lift up
  my hands and call on your name.
For you have been my help, and in the shadow of your wings,
  I sing for joy.

Psalm 63

ᴧᴧᴧᴧᴧᴧᴧᴧᴧᴧᴧᴧᴧᴧᴧᴧᴧᴧᴧᴧᴧᴧᴧᴧ

# Memory and Motive

As kingfishers catch fire, dragonflies draw flame;
As tumbled over rim in roundy wells
Stones ring; like each tucked string tells, each hung bell's
Bow swung finds tongue to fling out broad its name;
Each mortal thing does one thing and the same:
Deals out that being indoors each one dwells;
Selves – goes itself; *myself* it speaks and spells,
Crying *What I do is me: for that I came.*

GERARD MANLEY HOPKINS[1]

One Ash Wednesday I was asked to preach a sermon which
deliberately drew on my own personal experience of suffering.
The intent was not only to tell a story, but also to confront general theological propositions with actuality, either to challenge
or to confirm and illuminate them. No one can tell such a
story with anything but the utmost diffidence; but because
it was found to be helpful, if harshly thought provoking, I
was encouraged to publish it as an article.[2] In no sense
could, or should, my story be transformed into a "tidy"
or "academic" piece. Nor does it solve the questions it
raises; their irresolvability is the very heart of it. It is the raw
material of part of a life which both stands in judgement on,
and is judged by, theology. It is important that it is written by
a laywoman with no particular resources except the ministry
and the sacraments of the Church, and the particular ministry

1 "As kingfishers catch fire", *Poems by Gerard Manley Hopkins,* ed.
Norman H. Mackenzie (Folio, London 1974), p. 90
2 *Theology* (November 1985), pp. 441-6

of individual clergy and friends to help try to resolve problems. For most of us are like this, and these are the resources generally available to the laity.

Part of the pain of living the story of which I spoke in that sermon, the story of a mother with a sick child living on hospital wards, was that I could not solve intellectually any of the problems that arose for me. I was trained as an academic, but inapplicably for my new situation, as a historian. I sat helplessly exposed to raw experience, thinking and feeling that if only, above all, I had been a theologian, I could "solve" some of the more important questions that arose for me about the nature of the God I believed in, whom I thought to be omnipotent, yet who permitted all this innocent suffering. As a non-theologian, I felt helpless to resolve this tension between religious belief and observed fact. Intellectual helplessness was the least of all the problems in my personal desolation. But it remained yet another piece of human wastage. If only an academic theologian had been sitting in my place on those wards, I felt, we might be saved the statutory inept chapter on the suffering of children or animals in books on suffering, which so patently reveals that their authors had never in their lives been in the kind of real fix that I found myself in. The outstanding exception is the book by a Jewish rabbi whose son was born with a rare condition involving rapid ageing, who died as an old man, as it were, at fourteen. His father wrote:

I knew that one day I would write this book. I would write it out of my own need to put into words some of the most important things that I have come to believe and know. And I would write it to help other people who might one day find themselves in a similar predicament. I would write it for all those people who wanted to go on believing, but whose anger at God made it hard for them to hold on to their faith and be comforted by religion. And I would write it for all those people whose love for God and devotion to Him lead them to blame themselves for their suffering and persuade themselves that they deserved it.[3]

He succeeded supremely well except that he ended up with a powerless God, who is not responsible for "fate" and did not desire evil, without tackling head-on, as it were, the problem of a non-omnipotent Creator. In a sense what I am writing now is entirely redundant in the face of his work, except that I come out of an Incarnational and Eucharistic tradition. That Ash Wednesday sermon was my first attempt to try to formulate the raw material of my life in such a way that someone else could perhaps use it, and solve some of the problems that I could not.

I was astonished by the responses. The most surprising was that of the priest who had invited me, who turned out to have been expecting me to talk, not of my daughter's suffering, but of my own experience of physical pain born of the bone disease I have. It had never even crossed my mind to do so. One of the taboos with which many of us grow up in our society is a disinclination to talk of our own pain, in the quite proper attempt to avoid foisting it off on others, or boring them. And this taboo was one laid strongly on me in my childhood. I would probably never have gone on, after that sermon, to think of breaking it, and addressing myself to the other sorts of pain in my life, if the responses had not been so warm. People seemed to find the very breaking of the taboo had been of use to them. I was encouraged to publish the sermon, and was then startled by the letters people wrote. These seemed to say that it was the very honesty of what I had said, my very inability to find a neat conclusion, or to present a package, my very confession of confusion and bewilderment, which had helped them. The lady whose letter is probably

3 Harold S. Kushner, *When Bad Things Happen to Good People* (Pan, London 1981), p. 12

really responsible for this book wrote of the comfort I had
brought her because I had shared my "experiences, questions
and feelings, so that I may, if I can, hold on to it when times
are bad, remember your writing, and know that I am not alone
in confusion, and not lost".

I put that letter away. I put away, also, the letter suggesting
I should expand the article into a book on suffering. Almost
immediately after the article had appeared in 1985, we as a
family were faced with a fresh physical crisis. Our daughter
had to make a choice over a second kidney transplant. It
was a time for living, decision-making and survival, not for
reflection. Moreover, I hesitated, and still hesitate, to expose
my family and myself to the nakedness the attempt to tell my
story would bring. I write now only because all the members
of it have separately encouraged me to do so. When I initially
consulted my son, who was then twenty-one, on this invitation to write more at length on suffering, he said drily, "Tell
the editor you are collecting more data". So I said "no", as
indeed I had said "no" initially to the invitation to preach
the sermon, and "no" to having it printed. Of all biblical
characters, I feel most akin to the unwilling labourer, and to
doubting Thomas, for here I am, trying to say "yes", just as
in the end I said "yes" to the sermon, and "yes" to the article.
But the essence, and the true value of what I have to say, was
all contained within that article, which is probably much the
most important thing I shall ever write. I fear to obscure the
relatively clean lines of it here, or to trivialize.

Part of my reluctance has also been based on a doubt
about the value of individual stories. People who seek one
out in trouble are most helped by attentive silence, into which
they can speak, assured of compassion. Any personal reflection of one's own is almost always destructive, or disruptive.
Yet since this invitation came to me, my attention has been
constantly caught by passages suggesting the possible utility
of such stories. Canon Vanstone wrote:

Experience, and the story of experience have meaning which cannot be distilled without residue into general propositions: but when it is, as it were, let loose among general propositions, it acts as a powerful catalyst and/or illumination, exposing dark corners, and separating wheat from chaff . . . One longs to hear from experience "knocking at the door" of theology and demanding to be let in – not necessarily to challenge theological propositions but also to illuminate or confirm them.[4]

There is a notable passage in Rowan Williams's *Resurrection*:

. . . we might say that the community lives in the exchange, not simply of charisms in Paul's sense, but of *stories*, of memories. My particular past is there, in the Church, as a resource for my relations with my brothers and sisters – not to be poured out repeatedly and promiscuously, but as a hinterland of vision and truth and acceptance, out of which I can begin to love in honesty. My charism, the gift given me to give to the community, is my *self*, ultimately; my story given back, to give me a place in the net of exchange, the web of gifts, which is Christ's Church. My self is to be given away in love, not because it is worthless, but because it is supremely precious, given to me by the hand of God as he returns my memory. Out of my story, the Spirit of the risen Jesus constitutes my present possibilities of understanding, compassion and self-sharing. My identity as lover in the community is uniquely coloured by the loves in which I have already struggled, failed, learned, repented: they are the reason for my present love being in this "key" or "mode" rather than that, the irreducible particularity of my gift.[5]

4 Personal communication
5 Rowan Williams, *Resurrection* (London 1982), pp. 43-4

If my story could indeed be a gift of love to anyone in need, it has begun to seem to me that I should try to tell it, above all as a thank-offering, if it might bring hope. For it has been a story of personal limitation and failure, and on occasion destitution, that has seemed at times totally outside my capacity to resolve or surmount. And yet by some persisting miracle of grace, the memories of the past, and the pain of the present, do prove capable of healing or at least of transformation. I cannot comprehend the process, but I am sometimes overwhelmed by wonder at it and thanksgiving for it. If it is so for me, then I do not believe there can be anyone else for whom it cannot be so, for my own limitations are very great. My circumstances have been in some ways so unpropitious, it seemed at times so improbable that anything worthwhile could be brought out of all this pain, that I am not infrequently filled by amazement and gratitude that anything constructive could emerge from such unpropitious beginnings, and roots so damaged. That thanksgiving seems to need a voice.

*

If memory is to be searched, because we find ourselves accepted after all in the pain of it, and can therefore perhaps help other people accept their memories, and their own value too; if we find that that kind of truth can indeed "be assimilated into a present experience of gratitude, affirmation, praise"[6] in the presence of God, then a further problem arises. How on earth is such truth to be arrived at? It is not the problem of a prude: truth may be a naked lady, but there are worse things than undress – above all, untruth. It is more inability. Even St Augustine was infuriated by his inability to get at something as relatively simple as his own motive for stealing pears.

6 Rowan Williams, *op. cit.*, pp. 36-7

18

What is the truth of it? Who shall show me, unless He that illumines my heart and brings light into its dark places? What is the thing that I am trying to get at in all this discussion?[7]

Even with as total a conscious commitment to candour as possible, even in the presence of a good psychotherapist, or a good priest whom one trusts, even given determination to co-operate with healing, or with grace, it is still possible to stumble to a halt, not knowing the truth of one's own motives. All one can do is to be as transparent as possible, admit the uncertainties, and reflect on the suggestions made by such a person that ring true, or half-true.

In what I have written here I have tried to be as truthful as possible. Some areas I have avoided altogether, but I have written nothing that I knew, or suspected, to be false. Some of my motives must be unknown to me. I know very well of the persistent wrestling match that has seemed to go on all my life, as I have tried to make sense of the actions of a loving God who permitted such hurt. It is natural to me to try to solve such dilemmas on paper. I know also of the desire to be of use, in itself perhaps suspect, because it must be compensatory for the isolation which unusual experience brings. But there must be other less creditable motives: the catharsis of expressing such intolerable experience, which at times seems to take up all one's mind, is one. Pain has its own pressure. There is a need to do something with it, to make it a medium, and give it a voice. If I could do anything but write prose, I would try to make music with it, since music does what I am trying to do. But I am not a composer. I listen to the slow music of Mozart's clarinet concerto over and over again, because it seems to harmonize opposites, and state paradox, and says what I want to say.

7 St Augustine, *Confessions*, II, VIII. I have used the translation by F.J. Sheed (London, reprinted 1987) throughout

Of my motives for writing this story down, the account that rings most true would be that I would like it to make music.

I could be accused of self-justification, since I have not always agreed with the suggestions of modern medicine. I do not think this is right, although it does contain a truth, since I feel much more like someone engaged in a dialogue which has no "right" answer, but in which both protagonists must speak and respect each other's opinions.[8] But it seems a possibility. Last of all, there is the possibility of smug self-gratification of the crude "Just look what I've done and where I started from!" kind. Is the whole thing some vast egotistical exercise? I am indeed amazed that out of the confusion of my own reality anything of value seems to have emerged, but if it has, it does not feel as if I were responsible, rather as if, despite the poor quality of the canvas, the Artist had managed to say something after all.

*

At first sight a book which is about physical or mental pain may seem very oddly titled *Celebration*. But it is written by a woman to whom, over the years, participation in the Eucharist has become the most important part of living, and being in silence before the reserved sacrament the most important part of prayer. Gradually, and with immense diffidence, I have come to see that my own participation in this offering of the Eucharist[9] must involve the presentation of my own experience, for hallowing, along with "the best bread that can conveniently be gotten", in the hope that it, too, can be redeemed and transformed. Becoming a Benedictine oblate fifteen years ago seemed just a logical extension of this

8 See below, especially pp. 114-15
9 All this is said properly by Dom Gregory Dix, *The Shape of The Liturgy* (London 1943), and condensed on pp. 247-8

procedure at the Offertory. The presentation at the Offertory is re-affirmed in the post-Communion prayer, which is so terrifying in its total implications. "Here we offer and present to you, O Lord, ourselves, our souls and bodies, to be a reasonable, holy, and living sacrifice." Much of the experience I have had to offer has been untidy and messy. A great deal of it has seemed to me to be purely evil,[10] and as such, to make an extremely dubious offering, which at times was all I had. This private offering of mine has been deformed, and incomplete: I have been glad that if I was indeed part of the Body of Christ, the other members were bound to be making a better job of it. If I here concentrate on the evil, the pain, and the "wrongness" of creation as I have experienced it, I do so knowing that my initial emphasis is inevitably distorted.

I am also up against the barriers of language. It is much more possible for me to describe the experience of pain than it is for me to describe the ways it is capable of transformation. Perhaps we all find it easier to describe Good Friday than our own experience at Easter. It is probably impossible to convey that in the living-out they can sometimes, somehow, be one event. If I were a poet, or a musician, perhaps I would have the resources. But if Dante's *Purgatory* was more forcible than his *Paradise*, even this seems very unlikely. Even painters cannot, with the possible exception of Fra Angelico, paint Heaven. Hell, or the fear of it, comes more easily off the brush. Three and a half of the four walls of fourteenth-century frescos by the significantly titled Master of the Triumph of Death in Pisa, are given over to Death, Judgement and Hell: only half a wall attempts Paradise, and that is strangely inept. I was reminded of that constrained and lame attempt in Pisa, when my husband and I were standing in front of a magnificent Flemish Last Judgement that had ended up in Danzig. The souls to our Lord's left

10 I do not intend to engage at all with the problem of whether evil exists, or is "merely" the absence of good

in their descent to damnation were vivid enough: but the blessed to his right were curiously inert, smug at best. Our guide said suddenly, "It's odd, isn't it, how the blessed always look as if they had been *stuffed*?" I was reminded of that conversation when I talked to a historian of the *Annales* school, who had not only observed the phenomenon, but of course, being French, quantified it. According to him, the overwhelming majority of 350 illustrations in the Office for the Dead in fifteenth-century Books of Hours concentrated on pain and damnation: there was very little attempt to convey salvation or delight. He did tell me, though, that musicians could, and did, in settings for Easter week, make this attempt successfully. It is not an attempt I can make: here, indeed, I am deliberately focusing on the negative, and thus contributing a little to an unbalance I actually loathe. If I attempt to rectify the distortion in any way, there is a risk of travesty. How can I convey any of the perceptions of the sheer beauty of God that sometimes grasp me? I am forced back on to other men's words. The psalmist wrote:

I have looked upon you in the sanctuary, beholding your power and glory.

It came as a relief to discover St Augustine's capacity to begin to express the inexpressible.

O Thou, the greatest and the best, mightiest, almighty, most merciful and most just, utterly hidden and utterly present, most beautiful and most strong, abiding yet mysterious, suffering no change and changing all things: never new, never old, making all things new . . . ever in action, ever at rest, gathering all things to Thee and needing none; sustaining and fulfilling and protecting, creating and nourishing and making perfect; ever seeking though lacking nothing.

22

Thou dost find and receive back what Thou didst never lose . . . Thou owest nothing yet dost pay as if in debt to Thy creature, forgivest what is owed to Thee yet dost not lose thereby. And with all this, what have I said, my God and my Life and my sacred Delight?[11]

But he ended that passage:

What can anyone say when he speaks of Thee? Yet woe to them that speak not of Thee at all, since those who say most are but dumb.

This book is therefore bound to be seriously defective at the point where it matters most. It may be good at describing brokenness, but I doubt whether it will ever begin to convey joy. Without this, the Offertory is indeed incomplete and the thanksgiving never moves into the *Sanctus*. Not only is this a theological incompleteness, but unless I can succeed in conveying the possibility of practical redemption of the most peculiar circumstances, even of bare survival as a family when it looked impossible, never mind the laughter that has so often accompanied it, the record can scarcely be of assistance to anyone else. And in the humblest possible way, I would like it to be. Survival through the various ills that beset us was so wildly improbable sometimes that to give help to anyone else similarly beset would be infinitely worthwhile. And all I can do is to tell a story: just one authentic story.

*

The problem of bias in a record is one which I do know about professionally, and with which I am deeply familiar. This one is badly skewed. Because I am concentrating on the part of my life which has presented me with most

11 St Augustine, *Confessions*, I iv

problems as Offertory gifts, the story is slanted towards that of a sick mother with a sick child, and the way we tried to make that situation fruitful. It is also weighted towards the beginning of the story: recent events can never be so fully handled. My own creative work as a historian also has a part. My husband and my son, who are at least equally important figures in my story, deliberately appear only as shadowy figures in my margins. This is, in itself, a major distortion of the truth. A perceptive observer would detect the truth of the visiting close friend, who was heard to mutter, "It is good that a man should be Atlas in his own house". A student who spent the Long Vacations with us rightly dubbed my husband "the prime mover". Moreover, since my principal aim is to sort out what on earth God could possibly have been up to in this story, and how in any sense it can be supposed to be redeemed, I have left out all the details of time and place, parentage and circum-stance, which would be relevant in an autobiography. I have been, in brief, almost as maddening as the "spiritual autobio-graphers" of the seventeenth century, whose concern within their writing was the work of God and the soul, and who, in consequence, left out most of the material the historian needs to put their work in context. But my concern, like theirs, is non-historical.

# TWO

ﾟﾟﾟﾟﾟﾟﾟﾟﾟﾟﾟﾟﾟﾟﾟﾟﾟﾟﾟﾟﾟﾟ

## *The Beginning*

I have come into the hour of a white healing
Grief's surgery is over and I wear
The scar of my remorse and of my feeling . . .

. . . I have come
Into the time when grief begins to flower
Into a new love . . .
Now I have lost my loss . . .

In some way I may later understand . . .
And love I find has no considered end,

Nor is it subject to the wilderness
Which follows death. I am not traitor to
A person or a memory. I trace

Behind that love another which is running
Around, ahead. I need not ask its meaning.

ELIZABETH JENNINGS[1]

As the Irishman said, "If I was going there, I wouldn't start from here". If I was asking something difficult, I wouldn't have asked me. There was better human material available. The securities and tenderness of my childhood were shattered when I was ten. On a morning I remember as sunny, my mother came back from the bathroom and collapsed sideways across a bed in front of me in what turned out to be a massive stroke. The grotesque noises she made as I fled to get help,

---

1 Elizabeth Jennings, extracts from "Into the Hour" from *Moments of Grace*, (Carcanet, Manchester 1979) p. 7

and later, the picture of the scarlet, neatly-mitred, corners of the blankets in the ambulance that carried her away, stayed with me as unsolved, unresolved memories that I thought unhealable until very recently.

Memory may be healed, but the scars remain. That sort of experience is like fracturing a joint badly, only on a larger scale. My right wrist, which I once made a nasty mess of, does what is required of it, but although it mended well, it is not what it was before I broke it. The effects of emotional deprivation stay with you, just as would the effects of physical malnourishment on a child. A very large proportion of the healing process, it seems to me, is to come to accept, with some kind of loving tolerance, that that is so, that the deficiencies which frighten you remain, that you will never feel safe or adequate, just as your wrist will never quite move properly, but that you are still usable, and can still be used. But at ten, that kind of realization was far in the future. The next decade or so was a fog of misery. Anyone who has dealt with the aftermath and convalescence of a serious stroke victim will know some of the problems my family faced: my own were compounded because I did not know my father, since it was wartime. He now re-appeared, as a real figure, to find himself handling both these problems, and a frightened daughter. I had never been sent to school before, and this was a bad time to learn to cope with a peer group. There was a lot of illness in my life, some of it physically based and some of it not. The decade was not easy to grow up in, to live through, or to come to terms with. It left me with a profound fear of psychosomatic illness which proved remarkably unhelpful later, when I developed a disease which was physically based. Indeed, the identifiable beginning of the bone disease which has been such a bane to me was masked. My father died when I was seventeen, and I had to move house. During the move I fell downstairs with the business part of a bed and hurt my back. I put myself quietly to bed until I could move again reasonably freely, and told no one in authority.

In this fog, two emotional planks were provided that probably gave me all I needed to survive. Firstly, I had a much
older sister, who came home for the vacations, and provided
a core of sanity in the bedlam of tears and scenes around my
mother. Then when I was seventeen, just before my father
died, we advertised for lodgings for me, so that I could go
to school near this elder sister. The response to the advertisement planted me briefly in the shade of the household of
a Benedictine oblate, her five children and two nieces under
ten, and her other lodgers. It was a house of sanity and
laughter, full of life and love and warmth. From it, I became
acquainted with the parish Eucharist for the first time, and
decided to be confirmed. After it, I was old enough to seek
proper professional help for the misery, and was fortunate
enough to find a good psychotherapist. For the first time since
that sunny day my childhood was shattered, acceptance
became a reality, and it seemed possible to be loved. Indeed I
was loved: my academic work had taken off, and through it I
met the young man who became my husband, who above all
was characterized by loving tolerance, and a strong sense of
the ridiculous, which he needed. My life, too, became one of
love and laughter and work into which I could put my heart.
There is a real sense in which it is totally inappropriate for me
to talk of pain: I am so deeply fortunate in my marriage and
my work that concentration on the negative is, as I have said,
distortion.

But as I have also said, early experience is inescapable. The
scars grow fainter, but are visible. "We come to discover that
the moments of agony . . . are likewise permanent. With such
permanence as time has."[2] I learnt very early in my growing
that the unimaginable worst could happen to me. It had
already. No human agency was responsible for my mother's
stroke: at that time, I had no God to blame. Later, I knew, of my

---

2 T.S. Eliot, "East Coker" in *Four Quartets*, pp. 39-40. I have used the
  Faber edition (London 1970)

own knowledge, that belief and trust in a personal loving God was no insurance policy against disaster, before I even started on the pilgrimage I have found so difficult. At least, I was never lumbered with the kind of superficial trust that suggests "bad things never happen to good people", and never had to break through that particular set of clichés. It is difficult for me to say the wonderful trusting Compline psalm, as indeed it must have become totally impossible in the Holocaust, and maybe some while before in the Babylonian Exile.

For He will deliver you from the snare of the fowler and from the deadly pestilence; he will cover you with his pinions, under his wings you will find refuge; his faithfulness is a shield and buckler.

You will not fear the terror of the night, nor the arrow that flies by day, nor the pestilence that stalks in darkness, nor the destruction that wastes at noon day. A thousand may fall at your side, ten thousand at your right hand but it will not come near you; you will only look with your eyes and see the recompense of the wicked.

Because you have made the Lord your refuge, the Most High your habitation, no evil shall befall you, no scourge come near your tent.

Psalm 91

It is simply not true. God does not defend His people from worldly evil, and He seems powerless or unwilling to protect them. The trust one has to develop in Him lies far deeper, in the knowledge that He will be present in the deepest waters, and the most acute pain, and in some apprehension of His will to transform these things. No cheap belief in Him as "insurance" will serve. It seems to me that I came to this knowledge too young. It was, and is, a very important advantage, as I have already said, but it was double-edged. It is not good to know too early that the unimaginable worst can happen to one. It is difficult to see that decade as a source of richness: the only asset of which I am aware is that when people tell me of their grief and problems, as they sometimes do, there is never any temptation to judge. I have always been in a worse muddle myself. I do not think there is anything that can shock, or surprise, me very much. Nor is there anything I am afraid to hear. Meanwhile, my attendant demon is still fear. If one's spiritual journey is from fear to trust, I still have far to travel. To put oneself trustingly into the hands of God, when one knows His power to break, or allow one to be broken, is difficult. My daughter showed me a prayer in the book given to her for her Confirmation recently, which spoke to my condition: "Let us accept that we are profoundly loved, and need never be afraid." But it is a very long road to perfection in love.

# THREE

∿∿∿∿∿∿∿∿∿∿∿∿∿∿∿∿∿∿∿∿

## *Bones, I*

If I say, let only darkness cover me and the light about me be night, even the darkness is not dark to you, the night is bright as the day, for darkness is as light with you.

For you formed my inward parts, you knitted me together in my mother's womb. I praise you for you are fearful and wonderful, wonderful are your works.

You know me right well, my frame was not hidden from you when I was being made in secret, intricately wrought in the depths of the earth.

Your eyes beheld my unformed substance, in your book were written, every one of them, the days that were formed for me when as yet there were none of them.

Psalm 139

The three years after my marriage were halcyon, not merely by contrast with what came before and after, and in some fuzzy golden retrospect that never was, but in the living. If I could indeed paint Paradise, I would be sitting again among the trees of a meadow full of oxslips, feeding my first-born child a few days old. Only now, somehow, that meadow is also the meadow full of flowers painted by van Eyck in the Adoration of the Lamb, and all my imagery

30

is fused into one perfect landscape. It is always April or May.

It was, in reality, a very happy time. My work had begun to take shape: I had had the idea for the book which I later called *Contrasting Communities* on the way to an adult evening class, with the baby stuffed under the seat in a carrycot, and we arrived shockingly late in consequence. Once I sorted out my own priorities, and decided to be a "working" mother for two or three hours in the mornings, and bring up our child for the rest of the time, I must have lived as perfect a life as was possible for me.

There were the first grumbles of thunder in the distance, though. I had slipped on a loose mat when we were six months married, and caught my spine on the clip which held the hose of the washing machine. This was more disabling than my similar adventure with the bed had been: I fractured a transverse process, and was said to have slipped both the adjacent discs. For the next six weeks I was kept flat on my back, this time strictly by authority. I began to learn about pain, and about working upside-down. I also began to learn about orthopaedic clinics. In that part of the world, they never took less than four hours, and often six: there were the beginnings of learning to accept passively what hospitals did to you, the beginnings of learning that "a patient" has no time of value, and therefore by a paradox is bizarrely given a bonus of unplanned time while he or she waits. That bonus of time, I began to perceive, even as I fretted, could be a godsend. Meanwhile, we thought no evil.

We got through the pregnancy that followed with the aid of the first of a long series of revolting-looking orthopaedic corsets, shaped in canvas and bone, or metal, or pink plastic, that were supposed to be moulded to the human form, but never seemed quite "me". The lady who stopped me and said, "Excuse me, I think you've put on a coat-hanger with your dress", had a point. When later I graduated to plaster casts, I was infuriated to discover that medical disregard for female vanity, or even proper feeling, was so sublime that I could be put into a plaster cast with only one hump in front, like an Arabian camel.

When I was seven months pregnant, I went down to collect some documents in Cambridge: as I waddled to and fro in my corset, I developed a pain in my foot. It became tiresome enough to mention at my next routine orthopaedic clinic. I returned from that clinic, which I had attended for slipped discs, with a leg in plaster for a fatigue fracture. "Oh," said the orthopaedic surgeon, "that is very interesting . . . they were first diagnosed during the First War, putting office clerks into boots and sending them on route marches, you know." But my husband, for once, was not amused, though I was taken by the absurdity. We still thought no evil.

Evil held off long enough for us to discover the profound satisfaction of being parents, and for me to experience the joy of that day in the meadow gilded with oxslips. There was one full blown thunderstorm then, however. As I fed our son, and we delighted in him, the pain in my back, which should by now have eased, increased. He was born in April; by June the constant jabs of pain up my spine were getting frightening. This phase came to a close on the day of our son's baptism at a parish Eucharist in Cambridge. I had pushed on through increasing pain to prepare food the day before, but, walking up the stairs with coffee in the morning, I was suddenly transfixed. I owe a lot to our son's godfather, who was fast enough to catch me before I fell backwards down the stairs. I had to miss the baptism. That week saw my induction into adult grief, as I lay in hospital with ten pound weights slung on to each foot, being treated for slipped discs, and facing the physical loss of the baby, whom I was now not allowed to feed. Our situation was made more complex because we lived in two places. From October to June we worked in the University of Keele. From July to September we worked in Cambridge, where our research material was. It was apparently quite impossible for different regional hospital boards to exchange X-ray plates, so it was not possible for the new team of orthopaedic surgeons to look at the earlier plates taken after the accident, before my pregnancy, to compare with those now taken after four months' breast-feeding. An earlier diagnosis would probably not have helped. But it did all add to our sense of confusion.

I now graduated to wearing a plaster cast. I remember at some point that summer seeing a girl come out of a doorway, and bend over a pram to pick up her baby. She was wearing a yellow dress. I think I cried, for that picture of normality that I had temporarily lost, that simple shining ability to do obvious bodily things, in which I had so recently learned to delight. For I could not yet pick up our baby.

However, the world stabilized, and the storm blew away. In due season, I was released from plaster. I still was not allowed to lift our son, so things were complex domestically. We lived in a patchwork of domestic help we could not afford, and helpful students. Mercifully, our son was a fast learner. As soon as he had learned to climb on to my knee, and next to climb steps and stiles, the world was ours to play with. The halcyon days were back. In the mornings I worked, and in the afternoons our son and I walked in the woods, paddled in small streams, and cooked extraordinary meals. That was the longest stretch of external peace ever. If it wasn't April or May, the woods were always golden in October, and the trees all reflected in the lakes. The landscape that was going to be my lifeline in long stretches of isolation began to delight me.

*

But time moved on, even in Arcadia. We both wanted four children, and there was no reason why we should not have them, the orthopaedic surgeon said, providing I could submit to the indignity of being done up like a parcel in his pink corsets, and go to his clinics regularly. So three years almost to the day after the birth of our son, our daughter was born. It had not been an entirely easy pregnancy: she wanted to get lost, but we wanted her existence even more, and meddled with her plans. Under gynaecologist's instructions this time, I spent something like three months in bed, avoiding spontaneous abortion. There were more mumblings of thunder too, but still in the distance, not yet articulate. Late in the pregnancy, the jabs of pain up my spine started again; sometimes they were powerful enough to still me into immobility. On one horrifying occasion like this, actually on my way to the ante-natal clinic driving the old Bedford van we owned, for safety's sake I was forced to pull out of the traffic through a crash barrier into some roadworks. "Jhasus Christ, lady!" said the Irish navvy who lumbered over at a trot like a rhinoceros to point out the error of my ways in a flood of language I was too shaken to sort out, "Jhasus Christ!" And then he peered at me, and changed his tune. "I'm thinking I'd be better getting you to the Maternity." He seemed much too big even to squeeze sideways into the cab of our ton and a half van. Bulldozers were more his size. But his tenderness moved me oddly. There seems to be a particular compassion associated sometimes with very big men.

One can never concentrate on one's second-born in quite the way one can on one's first: the need to make sure the first is not excluded gets in the way. Also, I was suddenly pulled in as an emergency examiner to mark university final examinations when our senior lecturer died in the middle of the marking. The length of time it took to read and assess one question on a script, and the length of the baby's feeding-time did not quite coincide, and I always seemed to be starting a question again, to make sure that I was doing justice to the candidate. However, that passed too. Then came a magic day when I took our daughter into the woods by the lakes, and sat on a stone, and was free to concentrate on this new human being. It was early May; all the leaves were resurrection green, and this time the bluebells were out.

But now the storm would hold off no more. The pattern

of increasing pain that had followed the birth of our son re-asserted itself, though this time even more powerfully. Orthopaedic corsets were no longer adequate. In July we were on holiday in a cottage in the woods above the Wye, miles from anywhere, on our way to Cambridgeshire. I was facing pain of an order new to me. One day, when my husband had to leave me in order to help with an essential series of interviews, I was walking up the stairs with the baby in my arms and the three-year-old holding my hand, when again I was immobilized by pain. I was terrified of dropping the baby. I was also terrified of making any sound, or showing any alarm that would shake the three-year-old's sense of certainty in his universe. It was eight hours until I expected my husband back. When I could, I sat down on the stairs, my son by my side, and told him all the fairy stories I could remember, and a good few that came new to me. I have no idea how long I went on. Astonishingly, in the end I heard the sound of the baker's van. The delivery man heard my shout, came in, and helped me on up the stairs. I lay on our bed, and went on telling stories. I could feed the baby, but dared not move again to get food for our son. I asked him recently whether his memories were as horrific as I feared at the time: whether the foundations of the universe did indeed shake for him. "No," he said, "I only remember you having lots of time to tell stories."

I suppose that was the beginning of a fight that came to take most of my energy and drive, to make a world that seemed "normal" and "safe" for the children, in the face of the most peculiar circumstances. I suppose, too, I was determined not to let them down, as my mother had – quite without blame – had to let me down. I wanted them to feel secure, as I had not done. I was not conscious of this, but I don't think, looking back, that I could have behaved any differently if I had been. So long as I could be *there*, control all signs of pain, go on telling them stories, and be an available warm mother, I thought things might be safe for them. I did not want to become unreliable, and I did not want to disappear.

Our life continued to deteriorate; although still feeding the baby, I was by now unable to move any part of me without a jolt of pain. Two days later, I was put into temporary plaster in Gloucester Hospital. "I think, Sir," said the kindly plaster-room-man, after I had been sick down his neck, to the orthopaedic surgeon, "this lady is not very well, and ought to be admitted." "So do I, Tom," he replied, "but she won't leave her children."

Bedford vans are very handy. My husband put an old door between the back seats, and, on this make-shift stretcher, carried me to Cambridge. The ridiculous asserted itself in our lives, as it does so often. He arrived too late to find someone to help unload me, so I slept in the van, perfectly comfortably, and was lying there, feeding the baby, who had been handed in for the purpose, when the milkman looked in at seven o'clock the next morning. "Do you know," they said up and down the street, "the gentleman in No. 73 keeps his wife in the van?"

But by now it hurt, really hurt, to laugh. Later in the summer, our parish priest, a very silent Franciscan, was heard to whisper to someone in the hall, on his way out after telling me a ludicrous story, "You mustn't make her laugh, you know . . ."

Things were not funny any more anyway. Now we were back in Cambridge, where at last it was possible to make a comparison with the X-ray plates of my spine taken three years before, at an exactly similar stage, after I had fed my son for four months. Suddenly, in Addenbrooke's radiography department, the mood changed. A quiet, unfamiliar, grey man wandered vaguely in, and looked at plates. "I think," he said, in the manner of doctors everywhere, who think of *bits* of person, rather than person, "I'd like a skull next. And after that, a hand." "Who", I asked rather tentatively, after he had wandered out again, without speaking to me, on my stretcher, wondering what on earth this had to do with slipped discs, "is that?" "Oh, just the consultant radiologist", said the staff, soothingly.

Before they carried me back home that day, I had been told they suspected something very serious, but could not inform us what it was, or confirm it, for three days. I owe a great debt to Tolkien. I had not the faintest idea what we were facing, so could not start to face it: I now realized what "indispensable" meant. It seemed to me that only with children this size was one truly irreplaceable. "Motherless" came to take on a new meaning. As I lay in the sitting room, and fed our daughter, or read stories to our son, and played with him, I considered this new meaning. All the rest of the time, not able to start coping with whatever the reality was, I read all three volumes of *The Lord of the Rings*, and did not reach the far side of Sauron's kingdom until the three days, and nights, were up.

"Osteoporosis" said the metabolist I had never seen before. Orthopaedics were over, except for patching-up. "Idiopathic osteoporosis. We don't understand the cause. There must be some kind of fundamental imbalance. It just means you fracture very easily, and the spine is most vulnerable, of course. Very common in old age. It normally starts at the menopause; very unusual indeed in nursing mothers. Interesting. I am sorry," he said gently, "you must stop feeding that baby immediately, you are draining calcium out. We will put you in full-length plaster and we must get you mobile as soon as we can."

*"There must be some kind of fundamental imbalance . . . Interesting . . ." "You formed my inward parts, you knitted me together in my mother's womb. I praise you for you are fearful and wonderful . . . You know me right well, my frame was not hidden from you when I was being made in secret, intricately wrought in the depths of the earth . . . In your book were written, every one of them, the days that were formed for me."* There was ground for more interesting reflection, indeed, than even that metabolist knew.

I do not remember whether it was on the return from that visit to hospital or the next, that the worst thing ever so far to happen to me, myself, happened. Ambulance men are the most patient, and usually the most skilled, of all beings. This pair had a misadventure. As they carried me in through the door, one of them tripped on the step. As he recovered himself, he trod on his companion's foot. They stumbled. They dropped, and then caught, me. I can only have fallen a couple of inches, but the effect was terrifying. All my reflexes seemed to go berserk in the pain. I, who so much valued control, was completely out of control. I was screaming, not even able to stop in case my son could hear. My fingers were clenched in someone's hair, the world ran amok, and my husband, who was there, was utterly irrelevant through the pain. He could not reach me. Nor could anyone. "She probably collapsed another vertebra or two", said the hospital on the telephone, apparently. "Just keep her quiet."

It was months before I dared tell even my husband, who was not likely to feel that I had suddenly been afflicted with religious mania, and knew I did not go in for pious or saccharine imagery, that quite extraordinarily at that moment of unreachability, I had suddenly been aware even as I screamed, of the presence of the Crucified. He did not cancel the moment, or assuage it, but was inside it.

*

Our apprenticeship was now over. Later that year, we learned new facts about this bone disease, so common in old ladies. It proceeded from a failure to deposit bone, or an ability to erode it too fast, no one knew which in 1967. It was likely to stabilize in me, if I didn't do anything stupid like having another baby, and I was likely to be able to live as I then was, until I became menopausal. After that . . . doctors shrugged their shoulders. No one knew and it did not seem very rosy. However, I was then only thirty-two. I had heard of the sacrament of the present moment: suddenly, making the most of all the "now" I had seemed to be very important. I had, after all, at least fifteen years of present moments to live before I reached this unfaceable future. Unfaceable, because the moment when the ambulance men dropped me had taught me what real pain was, and I did not, really did not, want to learn any more about it, ever. It seemed even more important to live in the moment, and never allow the possible future to leak in and damage the present, when a local newspaper later made its way into our house, wrapped around the rhubarb. It carried a blow-by-blow account of the inquest on a lady who had died not of osteoporosis, but of pneumonia after her thirty-second fracture, when her second egg-shell hip had broken during a journey to X-ray the first. I stared at this newsprint in disbelief. The really odd thing was I could not destroy it. I hid it where our son could not possibly find and read it. To my alarm, it disappeared from its hiding place, later to emerge again, hidden under my husband's socks in his top drawer. So we shared that too.

Meanwhile, as we gradually acclimatized, and learned all this, we were back in our university at the end of the summer, with me immobilized in full-length plaster, unable to sit up, and with instructions to get mobile as soon as possible. We had a three-year-old, and a six-month-old, and a cleaner in the mornings. We also had the only bad GP we have ever had: since then we have been amazingly fortunate. "Nonsense," said this man, unbelievably, "when I was in the Army, we treated osteoporosis by keeping the patient flat on his back in plaster." In view of the instructions I had had, I grew frantic to move. He prescribed a tranquillizer. The more I tried to move privately at night, and got into pain, the more tranquillizer he prescribed. It took me the whole of thirteen weeks, and eventually the threat of a letter to my M.P. if he could not make contact with Addenbrooke's, to persuade him to bring in the friendly local orthopaedic surgeon who had presided over my life since I slipped on the mat, and now said I might learn to walk again.

That three months was a period of living so intense it still seems a kind of unforgettable base line of experience, a touchstone against which to measure the rest. I learned something very important during it. I must somewhere have acquired some kind of muddled thinking about "counting one's blessings" and "looking on the bright side of things". I lay watching my babies, and listening to them, totally unable to look after them, and thinking "This is *not* difficult; I am *not* in an iron lung for the rest of my life". It took me a while to discover that I was actually stopping myself from getting on with living by trying to persuade myself there was no problem. Since then, I have listened to people who were similarly failing to face the actual difficulties that presented themselves. They, too, were trying to persuade themselves that other people's circumstances were more difficult. Of course, they often are. But a failure to face one's own problem, because one feels guilty in the face of someone else's difficulties – which can, by definition, only be imagined, probably wrongly – assists no one. If this story induces that kind of avoidance of their own truth in anyone else, it will do nothing but harm. One can only live where one is, now.

I was in bed in our only living-sitting-dining room, as I had been since the beginning of the plaster epoch. At first being there was accidental: no one could get me up the narrow, twisting stairs on a stretcher. Then we realized it was necessary for me to be in the sitting room anyway while I was bedbound, if I was to continue to be the main point of reference for the children, as we wanted. We had never wanted nannies, even if they could have been afforded. The merciful thing about a bone disease is that you are not *ill*. You can think, function, plan, work: you can do everything except perform the physical actions that you want. You can feed the baby, if someone will only hand you it, the food, and a spoon. You can work, if someone will hand you the work, and the pen and paper. If not, you must wait: they are already pushed enough to do everything that needs doing. You time your requests very carefully.

The summer had seen the introduction of a pattern that was to become familiar, in which I tried to work academically for my two hours, whatever the shambles that surrounded me, but was as involved, and as totally available as I could be, the rest of the time. The university workshop helped me in my own work a lot. It built me a special machine that went over the bed and adjusted to any angle. It was so solidly made that a three-year-old could climb up it and not tip the whole affair over. It had a perspex, slanted screen, behind which I could put three sheets of xerox of documents, and a clip-board for writing. The Professor of Geography walked by, and pointed out the obvious, which had escaped me, that felt-tip pens work by capillary action, so I could write upside-down. The ink flowed upwards. Now I could work on.

The main fight was to keep the world normal and secure, if we could. There were always odd bits of Lego in bed, and piles of picture books mixed up with the xerox of documents, and nearly-finished feeding bottles, and stacks of illegible notes beside me. On one occasion, after someone had taken our son shopping, and he had cuddled up with a packet of peanuts afterwards, next to his statuesque mother, the normal tickling in the middle of the plaster cast became unendurable. The patient district nurse excavated with a knitting needle, and discovered a peanut, wedged' somewhere dorsally. That woman was a saint. I feared her wrath when on another occasion my pure plaster bosom became soaked in the wreckage of a "chemical" experiment mixing colours, blue, green, yellow, red and pink, that somehow had got upset. But she only laughed.

More than one saint was needed, though, and was found. We already had a cleaner in the morning, a down-to-earth motherly woman, who loved our son and looked after him while I worked. "Never you mind, ducks," she said at Christmas, "I'll bring you a new spine from the butcher's." Although the district nurses and my cleaner were wonderful, the social services were quite unable, then, or until very recently indeed, to help. I vividly remember a social worker who explained to me that she could not go and put an advertisement in the local newspaper for domestic help, since this was outside her brief, but she would willingly take the children into care for me. I also remember a health visitor, at a much later stage, who came round after a long absence when I was actually ill with pleurisy. She had twenty-two months of back-notes to make up in her files, which were due to be inspected. When she had finished, she put down her notebook, and literally wrung her hands. "Sometimes I sit and *worry* about you in the evenings", she said. She was probably the first person to whom I tried to explain, short of breath as I was, that it is useless to try to imagine yourself into other people's problems. Apart from the district nurses, one of the few people who actually could do anything practical to cope with our problems was our bank manager. Once it had been explained to him that he would be keeping our family together if he did not bounce our cheques to pay for all this help, and, later, the constant train fares to Great Ormond Street that were a spurting arterial leak in our finances, he simply held the deeds of the house in Cambridge – and did not bounce our cheques for years and years and years. But what happens to those people who depend on the social services, not on the bank manager, and therefore get their children taken into care, rather than running up colossal debts so that the family can stay together? Our ability to stay together as a family has, in this sense, been related to our middle classness, I am ashamed to say.

I could not at this stage be left alone with the children at all. To give my husband enough working hours to cover the day we desperately needed more help. Into this extraordinary situation walked the first of the extraordinary girls who was to help us. She was Danish, one of three girls from the tiny Roman Catholic Danish community who became known to us as "the Great Danes". She had been sleeping on a park bench, jobless, in Copenhagen, when our S.O.S. reached her. She was square, and plain, and beautiful. She came into our room, full of the anguished tears of a three-year-old, and the howls of a hungry baby, and the impotence of a frustrated mother. Without pausing to take her coat off, she picked up the three-year-old and slung him easily onto one hip, and then picked up the baby and slung her on to the other. "I am Kirsten," she said, "where is the food?"

From then on we worked a rota: the cleaner covered the mornings, while the au pair girl was free. She took over at lunchtime, and my husband did the evenings, dinner and the nights. When something went wrong, like Kirsten going into hospital for six weeks, a group of students stood in: one of them is now amongst our closest friends. It wasn't easy, of course. The cleaner and I had already worked together for a long time anyway. The incoming foreign girl was learning to be the hands and feet of a mother she didn't know, who was determined to get continuity of handling if she possibly could. It was hard for her. For me it was hard too, never ever to be alone, never functioning fully, properly, but never off duty either. The duty to be disciplined, always, so far as I could, always to be even-tempered, and to make as few demands as I could for myself in a household so pushed for survival, was curiously exacting. Mothers are very busy people. Helpless mothers have to organize someone else to do everything they would do, and to do so tactfully, if possible, always watching the interests of the substitute as well. It got to be part of my code of honour that the au pair girl should get the academic qualification, or experience, she came for. Her interests became as important as the children's. I needed to get the balance of human interests, and needs, in my house right if I possibly could. I learned to lie and listen to noises, and to tensions: I got very good at inventing diversions. I also developed a bad habit of attributing any good new ideas I had to the au pair girl, or to the helpful student. The children needed every inducement to help them accept her as my substitute. I remember the shock when one student, more perceptive than the rest, said to our son, "That wasn't *my* idea: that was your mother's". I don't think I ever worked so hard in my life as lying in that bed in our sitting room for those months, planning, organizing, telephoning, diversifying, feeding the baby, playing, doing my own work, and completely useless. Years later, a piece of paper turned up on which I had had to write all the answers when I lost my voice completely with laryngitis a bit later. Part of it ran:

> The bacon ought to be at the bottom of the freezer: try turnips for a vegetable?

> No, you can't prove the existence of God by reason . . .

> Try the bathroom cupboard for sticking plaster. It *has* to be there.

> No, I *can't* explain the difference between an atom and an electron.

> I ought to be okay for a revision seminar next week, tell them.

> Why not go OUT?!

It was exacting, too, always to have a third party there, both as a mother and as a wife. You are just a trifle less spontaneous with your children if you are observed: you are a trifle more self-conscious in your marriage if someone else is, as it were, taking notes. The experience of being an au pair is a very important one, as I knew from my own experience. It is the first time you are away from your own family, and your own environment. It is the first time as an adult you can observe somebody else's marriage and family life at close quarters, and be appraising and critical, with no sense of guilt. You can work out how you yourself would like to do it. I remembered very clearly how I had formulated my own ideas on how I did, or did not, want to bring up my children, and how I wanted my marriage to be, as I had worked in France. Now I watched the eyes of my own au pair watching me, and knew she was going through the same experience. It was a little like being a glass-sided ants' nest at the zoo. For the girls, it must have been one of the toughest jobs they could possibly have had. As Birgit succeeded Kirsten, and Gertrud succeeded Birgit, we were enriched by their generosity and their extraordinary good humour. They gave us new customs, candles everywhere, Advent wreaths, special biscuits and open sandwiches. They took the baby to Mass. They gave us survival.

# FOUR

〜〜〜〜〜〜〜〜〜〜〜〜〜〜〜〜〜〜〜〜〜

# *Bridget, I*

Let in the wound,
Let in the pain,
Let in your child tonight.

KATHLEEN RAINE[1]

Now the dance quickened. We thought we were stretched:
now we learned that you always feel that too soon, and you
can, in fact, nearly always take a bit more strain than you think
is comfortable. The Lord may not permit you to be tempted
above that you are able: but you usually underestimate your
resources, or perhaps those He supplies.

The particular event which brought me face to face with
some of the apparently irreconcilable bits of Christian doctrine, and taught me to live to some extent in the tension at
the heart of a paradox, was this. When our daughter was a
few months old, it became apparent that she was unwell. One
of the experiences which we all have, I think, and which to
me is one of the most important reflections of divine activity
in our own lives, is the delight of creation. It does not matter
if this delight comes through cooking a good meal, or carrying out an experiment that supports the original hypothesis;
writing a sentence that both actually expresses exactly what
we want to say, and balances; or creating a pot or a picture
that works. There is satisfaction which is indescribable in
making things, which maybe comes only after months of

1 Kathleen Raine "Northumbrian Sequence", iv, *Collected Poems* (London
1956) p. 117

dreary slog. A minute piece of creation has "come right", and there is nothing quite like the joy of the experience.[2] Bearing a child substitutes for none of these things, but is greater than any, solely because on the parents then falls the vast responsibility of trying to see that this new human being grows up undistorted, warm, and able to receive and to give love.

I was horribly slow to notice how unwell this particular child was: all babies are sick and wet sometimes, and this one was just a bit sicker and wetter, to start with. When she got sicker than that, the same GP who had so often treated osteoporosis in the army, refused to refer her: when at last he did so, it was with a letter suggesting we hadn't really bothered to feed her during my illness, judging from the paediatrician's assumptions. Parents were new people in local hospitals in 1968. The Platt Report was not fully accepted. We hit an old-fashioned Sister, a navy-blue ship of the line. "Not much good you visiting her, is it?", she boomed, "if you haven't done any good with her at home, you won't do any good here." Our distressed infant, who was always thirsty, was put on a high protein diet and her fluids restricted. Five days later, she had a renal thrombosis and lost a kidney. The staff suddenly became quite polite. We sacked our GP. But I was still slow. Although I had put every ounce of effort I could into the loving and handling of this baby over the last few months, and always fed her myself, I could do so little else, and had wondered so often what the psychologists would make of being cuddled to a plaster bosom, that I really thought she felt herself to be Kirsten's baby. Initially I accepted what the Sister said: I didn't start to fight to be with Bridget until it was plain to me that the only word she could scream in the stress of a blood test, or a cut-down

2  As will be immediately apparent, I am deeply indebted to Canon Vanstone, not only here, and especially below on pp. 73-80, but also for privately and patiently wrestling with my incomprehensions on paper

to put her on a drip, was "Mummy!" Then, despite the Sister, I started to fight to be there. If Bridget wanted me, if after all I counted as her mother, I was going to respond to those cries.

It must be unimaginably difficult for nursing staff and doctors to imagine the depths of ignorance and shock they are dealing with in parents new to the experiences they themselves undergo all the time. I remained slow. The local hospital had no diagnosis. When they said her other kidney was "not really working", I didn't realize to start with that they were trying to tell me she was dying. It was not part of my set of expectations that my child should die. We know other people's children, even in Europe, occasionally do die: we read about it in the newspapers, and say "how terrible", comfortably. It still does not become part of individual parents' expectations. And this was true of me, despite the fact that in my own professional work as a historian I handled data on "infant mortality" all the time. So I was very slow to comprehend. When I eventually did, and took her to the Hospital for Sick Children in London, at something like six hours' notice, it came as a tremendous relief to have an Australian houseman say, "Look, you have a baby with one kidney gone, and the other crook ... I reckon we've got about four days. It's not very hopeful, but we will do our best." At least I could now understand, because it was not all wrapped up.

"Cystinosis", said the Reader in Child Health, who had come specially to give us the diagnosis, three days later. She sat on a low stool, I remember. Perhaps it is easier for them, that way. "It is a very rare, genetically-caused, metabolic disease. Cystine is an amino-acid, and in this disease, it accumulates in all the cells of the body. You see it most easily in the eyes and the bone marrow, but it is everywhere. We don't know much about its effects. But it is kidney function we know it does affect, and it kills from kidney failure. I am very sorry", she said, gently. "She will die when she is between seven and fourteen." In response to questioning later, she told us kidney transplants were irrelevant to us: the incoming kidney would be affected by the disease.

*

The time I spent in that ward in the Hospital for Sick Children was some of the most painful and formative in my life. The medicine and the support were magnificent. The problems lay in exposure to so many fundamental issues. Oddly, you only get any approach to Third World mortality in the most sophisticated wards of the most sophisticated hospitals of the First World, with, in this case, a national catchment area of the most intractable diseases. Children were dying, on the particular ward I was on, mainly of genetically-caused malfunctioning.

Now the existence of Belsen and its like, that is, of humanly-created evil, I could, as a historian, cope with intellectually. Genetic evil, creation malfunctioning from birth or from conception (as it was in my daughter's case), was more than I could account for or understand. These children suffered – and small children suffer very acutely, and worse because no explanation is possible to them – because they were *made wrong*. The evidence of divine activity in, and through, creation and the minute ways we share in it has always been particularly important to me. Now here I was, living week after week surrounded by the evidence of failed creation, the rejections of our heavenly Father, the pots on which the potter's hand did indeed seem to have slipped. I think the bottom came for me one day when I tried to comfort a tiny anguished child (words are useless, only touch will do), and as I reached to stroke his head a nurse said hastily, "Don't touch him, his skull might fracture". That same day a "pious" friend called, and said enviously, "Your faith must be such a comfort to you". It was not. Belief in an omnipotent and all-loving Creator who is capable of producing results like those I was observing, produced for me at least as many problems as it solved.

So there was I, a Christian, committed to the doctrine of a loving, omnipotent Father, a Creator. And there was I, living in surroundings which persistently denied this omnicompetence, amongst the "failures" of His creation.

That was the worst problem at one level. At another, much more profound, came my discovery of what really mattered to me about our daughter. She was a much-wanted baby. When I took her to London, I did so all eagerness to save her life, and all co-operation; it came as an enormous shock to discover about myself, in the days of intensive diagnostic tests that followed, that I had other, much less rational, instincts. I had never understood before why sows swallowed threatened piglets: now I discovered, as I held a baby who was increasingly only capable of screaming "Mummy!", that my instinct to defend her threatened to override my instinct to protect her in the long-term, and therefore to get a diagnosis. The violence of my reaction to my child, constantly threatened by paediatricians incidentally hurting her in the need to get the result which both they and I wanted, was so strong that it took me totally by surprise. My experiences at night in the parental unit, listening to other parents shocked by the same response, showed me that my own reaction was not unusual. For half of one night I sat up with a father who had assaulted a houseman. The reason was simple: the child was dying of cancer and in great pain, and the houseman had a syringe of morphia, which he said it was not time to administer yet.

After a week or two of this, it did not matter to me whether our daughter had three left feet, or even, very much, whether she died now or later. What *did* matter was whether she became emotionally deformed by experiences which impaired her ability to love and to trust. Her emotional normality was all I cared about by then. We were long past wanting her to live at any cost, for possessive reasons, because we had so much wanted this child. What was intolerable was watching her learn fear: her fluid and chemical balance changed so fast that it was adjusted on the basis of six-hourly blood tests. Sometimes these were intravenous, but most often, a laboratory technician dug a triangle of razor blade into her fingers. She had very small fingers and sometimes, not having enough blood, he needed to cut her again. She learned fast. I am never going to be able to forget the sound of her screams. Very soon the rattle of a technician's bottles was enough to warn her. At first, I thought it stupid that a doctor about to engage in some painful exercise should put on a white coat, since that too was enough to warn her. Then I learned to hope that she might only fear people in white coats, so that the rest of the world was free from all this association with pain. In a doctor's world these were small pains, not worth noticing, or even observed, but I learned to dread the monotonous, constant, routine repeat of them over and over and over again. Above all, I remember the occasion when, having failed to get into either arm-vein, someone held her upside down for the houseman to get into her jugular. That time, her screams of "Mummy!" were practically choked. I was so afraid of being thrown out if I showed my distress, and indeed could only support her by trying to remain a rock in this terrible sea, that I sat there through anything and everything – punctures to sample her bone marrow, cut-downs to attach drips to her veins, and all – saying over and over again, evenly and levelly, in response to her screams, "It's all right. Mummy's here". It was all, literally all, I could do. In her late teens, long past the age other parents had stopped being there, I sat with her again through medical procedures that I was afraid would re-awaken all those repeat experiences of her infancy. Indeed, on one occasion they did: somebody in a hurry produced an unsophisticated bit of razor blade, instead of a needle, to do a blood test when she was already doped with pre-medication. No one else knew why my daughter – who normally never even said "Ow!", and had not since she was about four – suddenly screamed.

This new set of experiences, living with our humanely

treated, routinely tormented, baby in hospital, give me the right to say from experience that the pain of one's child, or someone very close to one, is worse than one's own. I know, because I would rather have been dropped again by the ambulancemen. My husband suffers in the same way over me, I believe. It was because of those repeat experiences that, when we were told that, in order to maintain her fluid balance and chemistry, it would be necessary for this one-year-old baby to be maintained in hospital "for months, perhaps more than a year", I asked for her to be allowed to die. I thought I knew from my experience as a mother to our other child that there was no way we could bring out of that year a normally responsive child, able to give and receive love. Moreover, I had had the opportunity to observe plenty of "unattached" "hospital" one-year-old babies in that ward. They would go to anyone, with equal response, or lack of it. I also saw older children sitting in their cots, banging their heads, either because of their medical condition, or because they had effectively been abandoned. I was over-ruled. So all we could do was try to make what seemed the impossible, possible.

She was in hospital for nearly a year. We got her out, in the end, for her second birthday. A lot of that time I was with her on the ward in London, but for part of it she was transferred back to our local hospital, and retransferred to London when she became too chemically unstable, or too complex. One of us spent at least half of every day with her, except for one shocking six weeks when my back muscles gave up completely, and then my mother-in-law, who worked in London, helped.

\*

I have used the singular first person rather a lot during the last section, and this brings me to a very important point: my husband and I have nursed our daughter, and made a family *together*. Alone, neither of us could ever have managed. I have used the singular pronoun partly because impression and experience is so individual, but partly for a very grim reason. Although we both record particularly painful events photographically, as it were, we discovered only quite recently that the pictures in our mental photograph albums are almost totally different. One of the effects of nursing a child like this is that it is a profoundly separating experience, physically and emotionally – you are not sharing the same world. At least, this is true if you have another small child to be looked after, as we did, and particularly if you also live at a great distance from the hospital. It is also true if fathers cannot be resident on the ward. At the time, we were too thankful that I was allowed to be resident with the baby to feel like grumbling that we could never change ends, but we were not allowed to, with the result, of course, that I could never be with our four-year-old. So we were very alone from each other in our living through the experience, and in our decision-making too. My husband looked after the four-year-old, and I lived in hospital. Sometimes we met (but never without the four-year-old who could take in far too much of what we said) and sometimes we exchanged notes. Some of our biggest decisions were taken alone. The worst time I remember was the evening we were given the diagnosis – which, oddly, we *had* been together for. I could not quite bear it, and wanted to cry. So for fear of waking a baby on the ward, I stuck my head out of a window and cried, desperately wishing for my husband. In the middle, a night Sister came down the corridor and said, "Mrs Spufford, your husband just rang up and said he had managed to get a babysitter and could come down if you wanted. So I told him the baby was fine, and you were fine, and there was no need – why, Mrs Spufford, whatever is the matter?" So she set an eighteen-year old girl, who had been nursing for only six weeks, to look after me. But it was not quite the same.

It will be difficult for anyone to believe, but between the baby and me living in hospital, separated from my husband

and four-year-old for nearly a year, and then battling up and down the railway line, and then learning to run a gastric drip at home at night for the next year, and looking after the other child, and one of us earning a salary and doing a job, and us both looking after students, and getting our research done, it was not actually until six whole years later, when a beloved student whom we trusted with *both* children gave us a week's holiday for our tenth wedding anniversary, that we had any chance to sort out, and digest together, the things that had happened to us that day of the diagnosis. There is not time in marriage. Someone has to run a gastric drip overnight and organize the baby; someone has to cope with the distraught sibling, and make life "normal" and "safe". Someone has to catch the train up and down to hospital. And someone has to earn a salary and cope with normal professional commitments, plus, in our cases, both partners carrying long-term research loads. Furthermore we could never normally go to the hospital together with the baby, both because of the expense, and because one of us was needed to look after the other child. Unfortunately, reporting back to one's spouse is not the same as sharing the experience. I don't know how many marriages give up under the strain, but I get the impression from living in parental units that very many do. I only know that we were intensely lucky.

*

The sibling, or siblings, is the only part of the family unit more invisible to paediatricians than the parents' marriage. I have had support when I said I needed it for our elder child: he happened to be very intelligent, and the first crisis involving a paediatrician came when he was six, when he managed to ask, one traumatic evening, whether his small sister would live or not. We told him she would not, and he made a request to see the Professor in charge of his sister, to make sure (in our interpretation) that he was indeed a man to trust. Our son needed to check; and time was made for him to do so. I have never forgotten that depth of perception and generosity, which was very important to me. Later on, when it again seemed necessary, we received similar help for him.

Yet it remains true that I am still more profoundly concerned about our son than our daughter. In a sense, we have literally done everything possible for her. But whether we gave him enough security, whether we found enough time and energy to solace a four-year-old whose world literally came apart, is a more intractable problem. When I realized that our one-year-old daughter was dying, I took her to London at six hours' notice. Effectively, as far as he was concerned, I abandoned my beloved four-year-old, with whom I had a very close and happy relationship, for almost the next year. The time before our daughter was born, when I was doing my research and rejoicing in bringing up our son, still represents the golden age of my life. I have never been so happy. It has been hard to face my grief for the possible effects on him, as well as my own personal loss of parts of his childhood which I should have shared.

After we had the diagnosis, we faced two sorts of problems. The first was simply the practical. We had this baby, who could only live in hospital because she needed to take in over two litres of fluid every twenty-four hours. To do this, she had to be drip-fed at night, and constantly encouraged to drink measured quantities all day. All the results had to be charted, and the chart had to come out right. The nightly accounting was a minor Doomsday. When she was sick, as she frequently was, extra fluid had to be pumped in. She lost essential chemicals all the time too: so varying quantities of potassium, sodium, calcium, and so on, had to be poured in to compensate. She was to be kept on as low a protein diet as would permit any growth at all, so 150 ml of this fluid was to be milk. She was also to be encouraged to eat: not an easy task, since by now she associated food with retching, even if it didn't actually make her sick anyway.

Nothing could be done to get her out of hospital until

the necessary quantities of electrolytes stabilized, and she was not needing all those blood tests. We had a nasty proof of that when her chemical balance went wrong at Christmas, and she went into a rigid arc: that time British Rail held the main-line express for us, and the Hospital for Sick Children had a doctor in his own car waiting on the station platform: it was all high drama. "Tetany: too little calcium" was the verdict, and they carefully re-balanced her. Or was that the time she developed a drug allergy that gave her fits, and the next time tetany? I forget. I had never realized how vital chemistry was before. The Professor she was under was one of the few really great men I have ever met. He had the quality of total attention to the person, or subject, in hand. He also had an extraordinary combination of wisdom and sensitivity. He had two introductory first questions which might come in either order "Is she happy?", and "How are her electrolytes?" I had never known happiness and chemistry were interdependent like that. This was a man who was bold enough to speak of "building bridges between love and science".

It must have been sometime then, though my memory is foggy, that the local ambulance teams became accustomed, because of fractures, orthopaedic clinics, pneumonia and tetany, to beating a path to our door, like lab-trained rats. One memorable night, my husband opened the front door to a thundering series of knocks at 2 a.m. To his astonishment, a team carrying a stretcher rushed past him and started up the stairs. "Hey!", he said, "Whatever do you want?" "Emergency!" they replied. "Must be you!" and continued to climb. It took him some minutes to persuade them to go away, and look for the current emergency, living a few doors higher up.

Once Bridget was more stable, I was slow again. Getting all of this fluid into her was the remaining problem. It took the realization that she had actually lost vocabulary to push me into constructive thought. When she had first gone into hospital nearly a year earlier, I doodled for an idle hour as I sat with her. I wrote down all the words she chattered. Just before she was two, this doodle turned up in a pile of papers – she had lost almost all the words. "If nurses can run a drip," I thought, "why on earth can't we?"

"Ridiculous!", they said first. It took a very special senior registrar at Great Ormond Street to sit down and listen to the reasons behind my request. "I don't see why not," he said in the end. A patient Sister at the North Staffordshire Royal Infirmary trained me to put a tube down her nose, and we learnt the rules about fluid and diet. It was agreed that the ward staff at the Hospital for Sick Children should have her for a final month, to try to overcome her antipathy to eating. The month expired. A ward meeting was held, and the Professor asked the Sister for her verdict. "Sir," she said, "there are some babies you can coax, and there are some babies you can bully. Bridget isn't one of them. If anyone can manage her, Sir, her mother can. And she wants her." "Do you want her?" he said to me. "Yes please", I answered.

So, again, one magic morning in April, we brought her home, all ours to look after. We were back in business as a family, the warblers were just back in the woods, and the bluebells were out again. It was like being reborn. A month later, I took her to Great Ormond Street on her first out-patient visit. She had moved from her vocabulary of single words in that month, into sentences with nouns, and verbs, and objects, and to the beginnings of pronouns. If language reflects happiness, she shared ours. Her Professor summoned the ward staff for an impromptu meeting, as he sometimes did. "Listen!", he said, "this is like a psychologist's text book."

It was not all jam, of course. Being together again, all four, lightened the load immensely. But we did get incredibly physically tired. We had to get up hourly to check the speed of the drip. It was as well one of us had mathematical pretensions. You counted the drips, checked the speed against the second hand of a watch, and then fiddled with an awkward little plastic knob that quickened, or slowed, the flow. Then you counted the drips again . . . and again . . .

and again, and repeated the procedure until you got it right. My husband could *almost* do this in his sleep. I have always been arithmetically slow. After a little, I was counting drips everywhere, and estimating the rate of flow of the leaky bath tap in millilitres per hour. After a year, we were both so tired that we had not one, but two, repeater alarm-clocks standing in saucepans to go off hourly by the sides of our bed. Even they were failing to wake us up.

By the grace of God, a friend heard a little piece on the radio about a new machine that counted drips. I went back to my special senior registrar. "Far too complex", he said. "All you need is a pump. Much cheaper and much more elegant." He supplied me with a pump. This device had a front you had to take off with three screw-knobs, and replace in the same way. You also had to tie the plastic drip-leads onto the revolving gadget inside, with thread. The first night I tried to set it up in the room my children shared, I got dextrose solution on to my thread so it was slippery. Then I dropped one of the knobs into the nappy-bucket. As I ferreted in this, my hands sticky with dextrose, a cry of panic went up from the six-year-old, "Mummy, the gerbils have escaped into the garden, and the *owl* will get them!" One hour later, two gerbils safely cornered in a waste-paper basket in the garage, I realized I was going to have to keep our daughter in bed an hour longer the next day to sort out her fluids. There were other handicaps to being a nurse-substitute, as well as my incompetence. One of them was that the time I spent setting up a drip at night counted as time spent with his sister to one child, whereas to the other it was not time spent concentrating on her, but wasted on a tiresome nursing procedure. I swore perdition on elegant little pumps, and went back again to my special senior registrar. A month later, thanks to a charity, the miraculous machine that counted drips was installed. It could control the rate of flow itself: it could even blow a whistle when it broke down. We slept.

It was all transformed, compared to the hospital phase.

That same registrar was brave enough to visit us when he came to Cambridge for a conference. He said he wanted to see how parents lived. He came to coffee. We had got the children to bed, by some unlikely feat of timing, and the drip was safely running. It all seemed very civilized, and we had lit the candles in the sitting room. I had totally forgotten the gerbils. They had escaped too many times for me, and I had failed to solve their accommodation problem, so they had taken up residence inside the bottom of the grandfather clock, whence they sometimes ventured out, to wreak havoc on textiles. I kept on swearing I'd make time to do something about it. Now, in the quiet, they emerged, and slipped across the room in the candlelight, drawn magnetically by our guest's trouser bottoms. They perched incredibly symmetrically, one on each foot, unobserved by him, and started to nibble. "Excuse me," I said, thinking that to send him back to Great Ormond Street with scalloped bottoms to his trousers would be a poor reward, "could you look down?" He did so, and a slow smile spread over his face. "So *this* is how parents live!" he said.

*

The gerbils were symbolic of part of the solution to our other problem. At one level we were trying to solve all the practical business of living with a twenty-four hour fluid chart, getting it right, but not getting into a fuss about it. It was essential that our lives should not be dominated by this gastric drip and these fluids, but that we should live as normally as possible. I think we managed, thanks to gerbils and the hard work of our au pair girls, and also to the simple business of having so much to do that the drip fell into its proper place as background. We were helped by the lucky accident of my temperament over food, perhaps. I have always been careless, and relaxed about it: I never fretted if Bridget did, or did not, eat, and I did not worry too much about that drip, either. I do not think it even dominated her own life. We tried to keep the whole thing as routine, and low-key, as possible. That was not especially difficult for us. It might have been much more so, if I had not been writing up my Ph.D. thesis that year, and much too busy to allow predominance to gastric drips.

At another level, we were trying to live in the moment as fully as we possibly could. I had begun to learn to do that over myself, and my own time of active life, once I had inferred it might well be limited. The essence of the proposition we now had to face, after this second diagnosis, was the adjustment to bringing up a daughter who was, quite definitely, we had been told, going to die in her childhood or early teens. So all the luggage of parental expectations, of planning for a non-existent future, which we all carry about with us without even examining it (I didn't even know I had it), had to be disregarded. In its place, we had to adapt to a régime of nursing care which was quite rigid, but within which we could carve out a life of normality for the child, and for the family, a life of seizing every present moment which could be made good. And this proved very possible, and indeed a discipline which taught us a lot about how to treat the present of our other child, and how we should live anyway. But it was decidedly not easy, in essence, and also because all but the best friends flinched away. So we found ourselves in some degree of social isolation, talking about the weather a good deal more than we would normally even have thought about it. This was not a situation that could have been alleviated by any change in nursing arrangements or medical support, which anyway were magnificent. The stress lay in the nature of the situation itself: nursing a child who would have died without constant and continuous medical interference, knowing with accurate foreknowledge that she was going to die in a few years, and transforming this situation to a "normal", good, loving, family life that felt as ordinary as possible, given the nursing restrictions. It is an almost impossibly taxing situation.

So we are not talking of stress situations which would

be alleviated by a little better planning. They arise from the advanced state of medicine at present, and the near-impossible demands this makes on parents. But we learned to delight in the present. Even if the task was almost impossible, the rewards were commensurately large. Every "normal" stage in growth obtained by two years of nursing, every trusting response and warm gesture was perceived as a miracle won out of evil. She was a chatterbox from the time we got her out of hospital, but she was three-and-a-half before she had the strength and muscular development to walk. She had just begun with a playgroup. I shall never forget Bridget's first footsteps in snow, so precise, and so delicate. It seemed extraordinary that she could have travelled so far.

# FIVE

೧೧೧೧೧೧೧೧೧೧೧೧೧೧೧೧೧೧೧೧೧೧೧೧

# *Work*

You need not see what someone is doing
to know if it is his vocation,

you have only to watch his eyes:
a cook mixing a sauce, a surgeon

making a primary incision,
a clerk completing a bill of lading,

wear the same rapt expression,
forgetting themselves in a function . . .

There should be monuments, there should be
odes . . .

to the first flaker of flints
who forgot his dinner,

the first collector of sea-shells
to remain celibate.

W.H. AUDEN[1]

I do not have the faintest idea why I am a historian. I
work on the lives of people below the level of gentry in the
sixteenth and, mainly, the seventeenth centuries, the latter
being the first century you can really get at them with any
ease. It is a very strange vocation indeed, to have fallen in

---

1 W.H. Auden, "Sext", *Collected Shorter Poems 1927-1957* (Faber and Faber, London 1966), pp. 325-6

love with these people, as it feels, to be working to re-create their lives from the mosaic fragments of evidence that remain. It is a matter of always sticking with scrupulous exactitude to the ascertainable facts. I recently read a review of the work of Lucien Freud which almost perfectly expressed my own much less fully achieved aims.

> Clear and precise delineation of what *is* constitutes the essence . . . Freud is not concerned with approximations. His Cranach-like scrutiny is of an intensity uniquely his own. As in canon law or medical practice, there is an objectivity in his relationship to fact which falls outside the brackets of pity. This "particular examen" of corporeality, demanding humility, pride and superhuman hard work, is more akin to the activity asked of a trained legal mind than to that associated with the layman's idea of "the artist".

> The result of this hard work is a vision that is incapable of being dismissed or qualified.[2]

This type of single-minded precision is part of the discipline, and part of the respect due to these humble people of the past. Elsewhere in the review, the author speaks of the painter's "adamantine attachment to the thing seen".

I could never have been a historical novelist, much though I enjoy some of their work: to fill gaps with the imagined, or the fabricated, is impossible. I cannot even, because of this training, adopt Ignatian imaginative methods of re-enacting biblical events in prayer. Within this demanding factual framework, I am re-creating with love, and respect

2 Patrick Reyntiens, "Galleries: Lucien Freud", *The Tablet* (13th February 1988), p. 178. Mr Reyntiens continues, "It is this intensity which frightens us as we view many of the pictures, whose subject-matter almost precludes our being there to look".

for these preceding human beings, all that I can currently grasp that needs to be known, and can be known, of their lives. Vocation does not seem too strong a word for my passionate involvement in this work. But it is so very useless: I envy those, like doctors, who can feel they are ameliorating the human condition. When I was a student, I once thought of becoming a social worker, but decided sadly that I was probably better at the origins of King Athelstan's prayerbook, which I was then trying to unravel, so I had better stick to what I was.

Being a historian is an even odder vocation in a much longer perspective altogether. If you start, as a believer, thinking of the actuality of the Communion of Saints, you realize that you are trying to reconstruct bits of the lives of people who already know, a great deal better than you ever will, what their lives were really about. The whole thing becomes preposterous. There is a wonderful piece in the introduction to a book by the Abbé Toussaert, who wrote on Flemish piety in the fifteenth century. He was defending his doctoral thesis. But he was aware of a much larger body sitting in judgement on his work. He wrote:

> This work is not only put in front of my examiners, but is also in the presence of an invisible multitude of bishops, priests, religious and the medieval laity themselves: they know, at this present time, what was their strength and what their weakness: they have already seen their terrestrial history in the light of the Divine Presence, and their eternal end is ruled by the sole True Judge who knows all . . . and who also will judge their lives.[3]

It is not the normal phraseology of an English Ph.D. thesis. It would certainly startle the examiners considerably to be

3 J. Toussaert, *Le sentiment religieux en Flandre à la fin du Moyen âge* (1963), p. 487

put so firmly in their place in the hierarchy of judgement. It is a good piece to quote, for it never ceases to surprise modern historians, who are not generally accustomed to thinking in these terms.

So I do not know where my vocation comes from, or how it was born, or why the drive to fulfil it has always been so strong. Like Mallory, who had to climb Everest because it was there, I try to put together jigsaw puzzle pictures of the "unimportant" people of the past, compulsively, it seems, just because they *were*, and I need to find out about them. I am only sure of two things. The passion was not born as a "displacement activity" for my physical limitations. When I married, I went into partnership with another working historian, and the arrangement has stuck. Secondly, the passion for empirically ascertainable fact has something to do with my mother. My parents were both very able scientists, and she, according to their academic records, and to my father, the more able. She taught me during the War, before her stroke. I do not remember learning anything of religion at all from her: nor do I remember morality being plugged, although I suppose that it was. I do remember, however, her saying to me "Never fiddle with the facts, dear. The pattern is this: you have an idea, and then you go away and find out if the facts support it. If they don't, you must discard it, and start again. Always change the idea, never the evidence." I must have been about four at the time. I don't remember much else of her teaching, but I suspect it has been more influential than she, or I, realized.

Writing and pregnancy have always gone well together, for me. If I had had twenty children, my output would have been prodigious. I had already written my M.A. dissertation, perhaps fortunately, before I tangled with the washing machine. In the next year I completed my first monograph, the week before our son was born. Then I had the idea for *Contrasting Communities* and wrote part of it before our daughter was born. But it was a big book, and the rough workings were many. I owe paediatric nurses a tremendous debt: in admitting Bridget to the Hospital for Sick Children, they also admitted her mother and her paperwork. I must have been the Sister's despair, but she, and her successors, tolerated me. They also tolerated my lying resting by her bed, even though I do not know whether I managed to express the taboo fact that I was in a lot of pain. When Bridget was asleep, or old enough to join the hospital playgroup, I worked. I shall never forget one houseman who came down the wards and literally prodded me, as I sat by Bridget's cot analysing the subscription list that set up a sixteenth-century school. "I can't think," she yelled, "how you work in all this noise." "I can," I yelled back, "if *my* baby is asleep: only you have just woken her up!"

I did ask Bridget's Professor whether I should give it all up, when she was still in hospital at the age of eighteen months. "What did you do with your normal child?" he asked. "Do exactly the same with this one." I have never ceased to be grateful. One of the things one sees so much of is parents with a handicapped child who have "given up everything" for it. Sometimes they have had to, the battle to maintain life has been so strenuous. But when the child dies, or better, manages to take off and move away, they are left utterly empty and bereft, because the maintenance of that child has turned into their main, or entire, reason for living. I have even heard of parents who have called their handicapped youngster home, after it had begun to take root elsewhere, to give back their own purpose in life. Even though I cannot at present balance my daughter's need for companionship and care, and my own work, I literally cannot imagine not having so many projects in front of me that they jostle for attention. Vacuum is unthinkable. Establishing priorities amongst them is the problem.

I do not really know, considering it, how my husband and I have managed to do so much. He had the vital salary to earn, and all the teaching to do, as well as his research.

I only did my research, organized things at home, and was available. We tried to take our major projects in turn, because the culmination of writing a book demands total attention, and one parent was always fully needed. It did not always work out. Much later, in 1979, to my shame, I queue-jumped on my second book. It was his turn. He should have been finishing his big book on medieval money. I trod wrong on a step, and tore the ligaments in one foot. A fortnight later, I hopped wrong on the second, and repeated the error. There is, frustratingly, almost nothing you can do without literally a leg to stand on. My husband said grimly, "You had better write that book". He lifted me out of bed in the mornings, put me into a chair in our bedroom, and lifted me back again in the afternoons. In the interval, I wrote *Small Books*. But I would have preferred not to queue-jump.

I had slowed up a bit during the year of the drip. Life was externally against us. It was useless to plan any scheme of work at all, not only because the frequency of out-patient appointments varied so much, but because the frequency of Bridget's admissions was so utterly unpredictable. I remember on one occasion being in the middle of a chapter which was going well, when I had to pack a suitcase to go down to Great Ormond Street. A visiting academic was coming to see me. I had wanted to meet him, and was very much put out. "Tell him", I said furiously, and utterly truthfully, "I'll be back tomorrow, or next week, or next month . . . but I *would* like to see him." Sometimes I failed to unpack the suitcase, feeling it might be needed again so soon that it would be a waste of time. One of our most ludicrous episodes was brought about by one of these "routine" situations, in which the visiting academic happened to be more pertinacious, or more desperate, than usual. My husband and I were jointly commissioned to write a unit for the Open University. Pages of draft text were lying on the dining room table when I had to leave for London. This indefatigable man, an editor in a hurry, was not to be fobbed off by my disappearances, but ran me to

67

ground on a ward in Great Ormond Street. "Yes, I quite see", he said, looking at the tangle of plastic tubing surrounding our daughter. "You are very busy. However, we really do need that piece . . ." "Tell you what", he said, suddenly, "no problem, I'll just come up as soon as she is discharged, and move in, shall I? I'm a very good cook, so if I cook, and you just look after the baby and write, I'll type as you write, and I am sure we'll manage famously." We did, too. We have probably never written so fast in our joint lives. There was absolutely no other way to get our delightful house guest to go away.

However, despite all these interruptions, there came a wonderful long vacation, when my husband offered to take over completely at home while I finished *Contrasting Communities*. He and Gertrud, the third of the Danes, a Carmelite oblate shining with joy, pushed me out of the door to the History Department in the mornings, and refused to let me back in until I could write no more, at night. They brought me meals in plastic boxes, and thermoses of coffee. I wrote 45,000 words in the next six weeks: it was all just ready, waiting for the chance. That Harvest Festival, Michaelmas 1972, I took my typescript to church in Cambridge on my way to the Press: it wasn't a vegetable marrow to offer, but it was the best I could do.

All these practical disadvantages of constant interruption and inability to plan might seem overwhelming. They were a shocking nuisance, and they certainly did have one major disadvantage. Time and energy were so short, and freedom from physical pain so brief, that the time I did, and do, have has to be strictly rationed according to a fairly rigid system of priorities. In it, my family, students in distress, students I am teaching, and the documents which record "my" people in the past, have absolute precedence. Prayer came to join these three. There was never any time for secondary reading of other historians, of theology as it interested me more, or feminism as it blossomed. My work developed in a vacuum.

Were there also advantages? I think so. One was the converse of the disadvantages: at least I was never writing to suit a fashion, and my work was entirely my own. Much more important was the extraordinary richness of experience to which I was, totally unwillingly, admitted. An authoritative social anthropologist once said to me about the seventeenth century, the period of time on which we both worked, "We are very handicapped in two ways, you know: we cannot understand the meaning of chronic pain, in which they all lived in the seventeenth century, and we do not any longer understand the meaning of ritual." I opened my mouth, and shut it again. He was an acquaintance, and to explain the centrality of either pain or the Eucharist in my life could have been boring or embarrassing to him. I have thought about it a lot since. At one end of the scale of expertise, the acknowledged master in my own field of social history wrote a magnificent book on *Religion and the Decline of Magic*, which has as part of its conclusion that the need for religion and its accompanying rituals, or magic, faded towards the end of the seventeenth century. This happened in part because of improved medicine, and the coming of fire insurance. The latter may sound minor, but is not. Fire, and the total loss of every worldly possession as a result, was commoner than we bother to remember. At the other end of the spectrum, I recently listened to a first paper by a research student who had just read forty or so of the "spiritual autobiographers" who wrote during the seventeenth century. He had discovered that these people interpreted events affecting them according to the doings of an external metaphysical being whom they called "God". "An uncomfortable state of affairs", he commented, "which must have lasted at least until the Enlightenment."

Am I, I wonder, profoundly privileged, or profoundly handicapped, by being, as it were, an insider in the tradition of the lives of the people I study? I admit to being very grateful for fire insurance. God knows, I owe enough to modern medicine. Without it, if I was not dead, I would be in a state of continuous pain I prefer not to consider, when I can help it. But even with it, I am in sufficient constant discomfort to feel that I can readily comprehend the problems of people in the seventeenth century with at least toothache. Like them, I know from experience about infant mortality. My problems are not essentially different from those of the people I work on, and with. As for ritual, it is at least as integral a part of my life as it was of theirs. My problem is not to comprehend, but to avoid over-identification, or mis-identification. What may be different is that I do not regard the evils which torment me as punishment from the hand of God, or signs of His wrath. I do, though, share their belief that these evils may be turned to His purposes. I do not feel distant from these predecessors, or remote from them. It may be that this common sharing of a world gives my work some quality of compassion which I would like it to have. Empathy is probably the historical virtue I most value, although I try to discipline it as strictly as possible within the bounds of the given facts, which are my canvas, and my stone, and my wood.

# SIX

ぐひぐひぐひぐひぐひぐひぐひぐひぐひぐひぐひぐひぐひぐ

## *Pain and Prayer*

Oh Christ, who drives the furrow straight,
Oh Christ, the plough, Oh Christ, the laughter
Of holy white birds flying after,
Lo all my heart's field red and torn . . .
And Thou wilt bring the young green corn
The young green corn divinely springing,
The young green corn for ever singing; . . .
The corn that makes the holy bread
By which the soul of man is fed
The holy bread, the food unpriced,
Thy everlasting mercy, Christ.

JOHN MASEFIELD[1]

I am fortunate to have escaped even the fringes of the ancient belief that physical affliction is necessarily punishment from the hand of God. But post-Enlightenment or not, it is still common. I learned this during a night I spent with a mother in the parental unit in the Hospital for Sick Children. Her son had an incurable, acutely painful disease.

She had nursed him for two years at home, and had had hardly any help and hardly any sleep at all, since the child cried continually, and screamed if he was touched. She was much troubled about some event in these two years that lay appallingly on her conscience. Eventually she told me. After

1 John Masefield, "The Everlasting Mercy", *Poems by John Masefield* (Heinemann, London 1946), p. 77

eighteen months, one night she could not stand the scream
ing and the endless prospect of her son's pain, and had put
a pillow over his face, intending to suffocate him. She had
taken it away in time, but the guilt and the memory would not
leave her alone. (Never in my life have I wished that I had the
power of absolution so much as on that night.) I asked her if
she could not go to her parish priest. She was horrified at
the very idea, and told me why. The priest had come to see
the baby, and she had hoped for comfort. But what he said
was, "What sin did you or your husband commit?" So I
learned that we still needed a better-educated parish clergy.
But on that occasion, unlike the one on which our Lord
rebuked the disciples for a similar explanation of malformity,
God was not glorified in the outcome – or at least, not in any
very obvious way. The child died in great pain a year or two
later.

Some authors who try to wrestle with the mystery of
suffering feel that man-made suffering, surely most completely exemplified for us in the horror of the Holocaust, is
more evil and more incomprehensible than the sort of genetic
evil, fundamental malformation for which no human agency
can be blamed, which I had now been brought to observe.[2]
They may well be right. If they are, I am not entitled to write
of suffering at all, for I have been remarkably fortunate.
The suffering of Elie Wiesel[3] and Iulia de Beausobre[4] and
all the millions of people they represent, are outside my
experience. I have met human stupidity, and crass error
born of miscomprehension, but never in my life have I met
with deliberate sadism, or even deliberate unkindness. That
unspeakable world is closed to me. I can only speak of the

2 Donald Nicholl, *Holiness* (Darton, Longman & Todd, London, new ed. 1987)
    p.136. I have leant heavily on Professor Nicholl in what follows, especially
    his translation of Teilhard de Chardin, and his reflections on the Book of Job
3 Elie Wiesel, *Night* (Penguin, Harmondsworth 1981)
4 Iulia de Beausobre, *The Woman Who Could Not Die* (London 1938)

physical world I have come to know, the world of innate defect, deficiency within the creation, the world where the evolutionary process produces the whole and the strong: but also congenitally thin-walled blood vessels, defective bones, and malformed babies. If this is easier, and lesser, suffering, it is enough. It presents me with more material than I can contain, or perceive to be transformed, or even be transformable by any love. I was surrounded on the metabolic wards by the failures of creation, the drop-outs of natural selection. But the language of science, and of natural selection, and the language of theological belief in a loving, omnipotent Creator, have to be reconciled. Can they be? Here was the crux of my problem. These dropouts were human babies, with all the needs of normal babies. I am never going to be able to forget the sound of those screams. Of all the Feasts of the Church, Holy Innocents is the most intolerable: of all sounds after the crying of children, the most terrible is the crying of Rachel weeping for her children, because they are not. Except when she is crying because they still are. I cannot reconcile the images of tiny, deformed children with old men's eyes, in great pain (children who shrank from human contact because so often it represented more pain, the stab of a therapeutic needle which they could not recognize as therapeutic) with what I am bound to believe of a loving, omnipotent Father. I will not assent to all this pain as anything but a manifest evil. One of the commonest Christian heresies is surely to glorify suffering as somehow "good".

In three successive generations – my mother's, my own and my daughter's – I have known physical evil. Two of those three times it was caused by fundamental metabolic defects, and of those two times one was caused by an error in the genetic coding itself. I have searched for a theological answer. I do not believe there is one. Would, or can, any theologian produce any answer other than that we are here in the presence of a mystery, insoluble in human terms?

Teilhard de Chardin at least makes the attempt.

On a tree, by contrast, which has had to fight the internal hazards of its own growth, and the external hazards of rough weather, the broken branches, the bruised blossoms and the shrivelled, sickly or faded flowers are in their rightful place; they reflect the amount of difficulty which the trunk which bears them has undergone before attaining its growth . . . The world is an immense groping, an immense search . . . it can only progress at the cost of many failures and many casualties. The sufferers, whatever the nature of their suffering, are the reflection of this austere but noble condition. They are not useless and diminished elements. They are merely those who pay the price of universal progress and triumph . . . it is exactly those who bear in their enfeebled bodies the weight of the moving world who find themselves, by the just dispensation of providence, the most active factors in that very progress which seems to sacrifice and to shatter them.[5]

This is not enough. In an adult, perhaps, pain and sickness can be transformed. Even for an adult, it is not an answer one is ever entitled to prescribe to anyone else, without intolerable presumption, although one might well apply it to oneself. But a small child is twisted by pain and illness, not only externally and bodily, but internally, in its ability to respond, to love and to trust. Can we really regard these infants as reflections of an "austere but noble condition . . . those who pay the price of universal progress and triumph"? The whole being rebels. Why is creation riddled with pain? How far advanced does an organism have to be to suffer pain? How far down the Grand Canyon does one have to go to find the fossil of some little creature, shrieking in pain, that prefigures the pain of the babies born with genetic defects whom I have seen? Why

5 Translated by Professor Donald Nicholl in *Holiness*, p.136. Originally from Teilhard de Chardin "La signification et la valeur constructice de la souffrance" in *Le Trait d'Union*, No.45 (1953)

is suffering stamped indelibly all through creation like this, endemic everywhere? Peter Lippert wrote:

You have created oceans of pain ... and I cannot see how they were necessary to preserve your world ...

Lord, everything apart from you is plunged in suffering. You allow the sea of pain to surge forward up to the steps of your throne, to the heights of your majesty; and all that goes out from you steps at once into these dark, boiling waves. You yourself, when you wanted to descend into the world, had to plunge into this ocean of suffering that surrounds you. Lord, you created pain.

There are some who know everything, who penetrate even your great thoughts and decrees and give a nice, tidy explanation of them all. They explain and prove to me that it has to be just so and is best as it is. But I cannot endure these people who explain everything, who justify and find excuses for everything you do. I prefer to admit that I don't understand. That I cannot grasp why you created pain, why so much pain, such raging, crazy and meaningless pain. I bow down before your glory indeed; but I do not now venture to raise my eyes to you. There is too much grief and weeping in them. So I cannot look on you.[6]

*

The story of Job is the first Hebrew classic on suffering to present it in story form. Job is innocent, and is stripped of his possessions, his children, and his health, to test whether his delight was in them rather than in his reverence for God. He both maintains his innocence and refuses to abandon his trust in God. The eventual response from God evokes the wonder of the creation. A modern commentator has written:

6 Quoted by Ladislaus Boros, *Pain and Providence*, (Search Press, London 1966) pp. 68-9

At this point the tensions between his concept of the innocent sufferer and his concept of the just God cease to plague his mind, because God is revealed as present in his own heart, which is filled only with joy, with no room left for his own concepts and arguments. For it is noteworthy that God does not answer the arguments either of Job or of his so-called friends or of his wife. To have done so would have been to acknowledge that suffering is a problem to be solved and not a mystery within which we can be drawn ever deeper into the presence of God and of one another.[7]

But I am more arrogant than Job. I will not accept the revelation of God's glory and might that satisfied him, even though he would not admit that his own lack of righteousness had brought about his punishment. God's answer to Job, which amounts to "Did *you* make the creation? If so, question it!" is not an adequate answer to my questioning. At this point in my thinking, I came across Canon Vanstone's work, which has meant a great deal to me. He wrote in *Love's Endeavour, Love's Expense*:

Supremacy is not the relationship of the artist to the work of art, nor the lover to the object of his love . . . respect on the part of an inferior may be dictated by prudence; but it can hardly be justified by moral sensitivity. Superiority as such conveys no moral right to respect; in particular, superiority of power confers no such right.[8]

So the answer that satisfied Job is not for me. Apart from solving no intellectual problems, it does not break through to convey the presence of the living God within his suffering

---

7 Donald Nicholl, *op. cit.*, p.138

8 W.H. Vanstone, *Love's Endeavour, Love's Expense: The Response of Being to the Love of God* (Darton, Longman & Todd, London 1977) p.61. In the following section, I particularly use pp. 47-68

world. It contains too much of power, without accountability.

The delight of craftsmanship and making things has always, as I have already said, meant a very great deal to me, both in work and in childbearing. That was one reason why the experience of living with the evidence of failed creation, those human pots on which the potter's hand had indeed slipped, was so bad. I needed to worship a Creator deeply involved in His universe, not a "mere" grower of trees, however unimaginably huge, however magnificent, bearing bruised blossoms and shrivelled flowers amongst the good fruit. An uncaring Creator was unthinkable. Like Ivan Karamazov, I would hand in my ticket, I thought.

The beginnings of an answer, not to the origin of this evil, but to its possible transformation, gradually came to me over the years of nursing my daughter, of fighting for her emotional normality, for her power to trust and to love. To start from the least, and work up. I know in my own creative life and my research as a historian the way the work is constantly going awry; the documents point in the other direction, the evidence does not fit the hypothesis, the sentence structure comes out wrong – I seem to be fighting with a living organism, and I must be obedient to its own growth, and adjust to the way this minute creation of mine grows, while still giving it discipline and form. I even know that my own utterly unwanted experience of physical pain, and the emotional pain of nursing our daughter, which were in themselves entirely evil, have enriched my own academic work in a way that was unplanned and unforeseen. Those things which were amiss seemed to have been somehow woven into the fabric, not entirely to its detriment.

I know also the way in which the imperfect growths in the creation of God take on a strange beauty all their own. The twisted tree is often the one to stand and marvel at: it has been given something out of its twistedness. There is a new kind of beauty which is intrinsically painful, yet free from the grotesque. As for the twisted child, I had learned how every "normal" response, so hard fought for, was felt as miracle, culmination beyond reasonable hope. And above all, I have come to value the insight and wisdom far beyond their age – but not beyond their abominable experience – that these children sometimes have. My husband and I have grown also to value, as everyone should, all these stages in "ordinary" children, which too often are assumed. Canon Vanstone's descriptions of the creative process at work – in which what is created, being "other than" the Creator, has almost its own power of response and therefore something like a freedom of its own to "come right" or to "come wrong" – ring true to someone accustomed to her own minute engagement in creation. If this is so, creation's freedom of response logically leads to a failure of omnipotence in the sense of total control. I do not see at all how this works at the level of evolution, which is the cellular level I need to comprehend and cannot. But perhaps this is just my own scientific blindness. Does matter, at this level, also have its own power of response, so that it too can "come wrong" in the way that is so familiar to the artist? Can matter itself develop wrong, as truly as men in their choices? Does it, too, necessarily have its own freedom? In Canon Vanstone's argument, the loss of total control does not lead to a failure of the inexhaustibility of God's love, which everlastingly seeks to redress that which is, or grows, amiss.

> It may be said of the artist that he is always stretching his powers beyond their known limit ... As the artist exceeds his known powers, his work is precariously poised between success and failure, between triumph and tragedy ... We see, at the moment of lost control, the most intense endeavour of the artist: and his greatness lies in his ability to discover ever-new reserves of power to meet each challenge of precarious adventure ... The existence of evil must be seen as the expression or consequence of the precariousness of the divine creativity. Evil is the moment of control jeopardised and lost; and the redemption of evil

is inseparable from the process of creation. The principle is derived from reflection upon the nature and activity of authentic love ... that that which is created is "other" than He Who creates; that its possibility is not foreknown but must be discovered; that its possibility must be "worked out" in the creative process itself; and that the working out must include the correction of the step which has proved a false step, the redemption of the move which, unredeemed, would be tragedy. In artistic creation the artist wills both content and form: neither is fundamentally alien or resistant to that which he would create. The artist chooses, let us say, a certain size of canvas as suitable for a certain theme. But, as he works, this formal requirement, which he himself has willed, imposes a discipline upon his creativity. He is faced with the problem of working within his self-chosen form; and the solution to the problem must be worked out in the creative process. The problem arises not because the artist has chosen the "wrong" form but because he has chosen *some kind* of form – because he has chosen not merely to express himself but to do so in some kind of determinate way. This problem is present in all creativity, in every process of imparting oneself to that which is truly other than oneself: one must "find the way" in which, through risk and failure and the redemption of failure, the other may be able to receive.

In the second place, the principle does not imply that evil is willed by the Creator, either for its own sake or as a means to a great good. The artist does not will the moment of lost control, nor intend it as a means to the completion and the greatness of his work. He does not will the demand which that moment makes upon him – the demand to redeem it and to save his work. He does not will the problem of creativity: his will is to overcome the problem in every particular form and moment in which it may arise. Each problematical moment is unforeseen and unforeseeable: it arises because the object of creation is truly an other. The demand on the artist is to overcome the unforeseeable problem – to handle it in such a way that it becomes a new and unforeseen richness in his work. The artist fails not when he confronts a problem but when he abandons it: and he proves his greatness when he leaves no problem abandoned. Our faith in the Creator is that he leaves no problem abandoned and no evil unredeemed.[9]

If this explanation is theologically acceptable, it would do much to heal the irreconcilable clashes in my life between human experience, and what I am bound to believe. One of the most helpful things that was ever said to me was "The definition of 'Almighty' means that there is no evil out of which good cannot be brought". This I have found, extremely painfully, to be true. The fundamentally awry can perhaps never be made whole in this life; yet like the twisted tree, or the child's courage and wisdom, it can take on a beauty of its own. And in this transformation, the constant presence of an enabling God seems to me vital. My image of a Creator in whose creation there are mistakes not logically comprehensible may be true, but it has to be extended into the image of a Creator who ceaselessly, patiently, works to transform and re-create what has gone amiss, above all in His own entry into this creation to amend and redeem it. Some of this re-creation and patient transformation of what has gone amiss I can myself bear witness to. But if those theologians who assert that God is in total control of His creation are right, I cannot worship Him. Integrity demands that I do hand in my ticket. For I still cannot cope with the endemic nature of pain. And integrity has to come higher than anything else at all, even God, or at least my present perception of Him.

*

9 W.H. Vanstone, *op. cit.*, pp. 47-8, 63-4

The Book of Job may be the first Hebrew presentation of suffering in story form. One of its most terrible modern continuations is Elie Wiesel's *Night*. This is not story, but a brief, economical, eye-witness, factual account of the Holocaust, suffered by himself as a boy of fourteen and fifteen in the concentration camps. On his first night in Birkenau, he saw a lorry-load of babies being burnt.

> Never shall I forget that night, the first night in camp, which has turned my life into one long night, seven times cursed and seven times sealed. Never shall I forget that smoke. Never shall I forget the little faces of the children, whose bodies I saw turned into wreaths of smoke beneath a silent blue sky.
>
> Never shall I forget those flames which consumed my faith forever.

At the celebration of New Year's Day, he rebelled, unlike ten thousand others.

> Thousands of voices repeated the benediction; thousands of men prostrated themselves like trees before a tempest.
>
> "Blessed be the Name of the Eternal!"
>
> This day I had ceased to plead. I was no longer capable of lamentation. On the contrary, I felt very strong. I was the accuser, God the accused. My eyes were open and I was alone – terribly alone in a world without God and without man. Without love or mercy. I had ceased to be anything but ashes, yet I felt myself to be stronger than the Almighty, to whom my life had been tied for so long. I stood amid that praying congregation, observing it like a stranger.

Elie Wiesel did hand in his ticket. His integrity did demand it. But in the course of his time in the extermination camps, he both saw, and heard, without fully knowing that he heard, a much more profound answer to Job than had been

81

vouchsafed in the Book of Job itself.[10] In the experience that almost, but not quite, epitomized evil above all other experiences for him a ten-year-old child was hanged, as a warning, along with two adults.

> The three victims mounted together on to the chairs. The three necks were placed at the same moment within the nooses.
>
> "Long live liberty!" cried the two adults.
>
> But the child was silent.
>
> "Where is God? Where is He?" someone behind me asked.
>
> At a sign from the head of the camp, the three chairs tipped over.
>
> Total silence throughout the camp. On the horizon, the sun was setting.
>
> "Bare your heads!" yelled the head of the camp. His voice was raucous. We were weeping.
>
> "Cover your heads!"
>
> Then the march past began. The two adults were no longer alive. Their tongues hung swollen, blue-tinged.
>
> But the third rope was still moving; being so light, the child was still alive . . .
>
> For more than half an hour he stayed there, struggling between life and death, dying in slow agony under our eyes. And we had to look him full in the face. He was still alive when I passed in front of him. His tongue was still red, his eyes were not glazed.
>
> Behind me, I heard the same man asking:
>
> "Where is God now?"
>
> And I heard a voice within me answer him:
>
> "Where is He? Here He is – He is hanging here on this gallows . . ."

In the end, unless my image of a Creator had not been

10 I owe this insight to Harry Potter

capable of transformation, by the very words of the Creed, into belief in the truth of a Creator who had himself entered into his creation to suffer with it, and to amend and redeem it, I too would have quit, like Elie Wiesel. To the knowledge of the Incarnation, not to the image of an omnipotent Creator, I have clung like a limpet. On those terrible children's wards I could neither have worshipped nor respected any God who had not Himself cried, "My God, my God, why hast Thou forsaken Me?" Only because it was so, only because the Creator loved His creation enough to become helpless with it and suffer in it, totally overwhelmed by the pain of it, I found there was still hope. But without the Garden of Gethsemane, without the torture and the gallows, there would be no hope for any of us, overwhelmed in the present by pain. So the horror of Holy Week is the only hope of renewal of life for the derelict. For He whom we worship was made like His brethren in every respect. Because He Himself has suffered, says the author of the letter to the Hebrews, He is able to help those who suffer now; but not, in my experience, by removing the suffering. The beauty of the twisted tree is still brought out *through* its contortion.

For me, the greatest literary evocation of suffering and its redemption at an unpayable cost, at a level of pain where the unimaginable worst has indeed come true, and the victim has not been delivered, is the novelist H.M. Prescott's description of the death of Robert Aske, gentleman.[11] Robert Aske, leader of the Pilgrimage of Grace, died in 1537, hanged alive in chains from the keep of York Castle. The facts are true. The man died, tortured to death, at the end of the rebellion against the dissolution of the monasteries. His own motives had been almost entirely religious. The novelist writes, with a stark, pitiless gentleness, which is unendurable, of his death, his cause lost, betrayed by his God.

11 H.M. Prescott, *The Man on a Donkey* (Eyre & Spottiswood, London, 1953) pp. 688-90

And as his eye told him of the sickening depth below his body, and as his mind foreknew the lagging endlessness of torment before him, so, as if the lightning had brought an inner illumination also, he knew the greater gulf of despair above which his spirit hung, helpless and aghast.

God did not now, nor would in any furthest future, prevail. Once He had come, and died. If He came again, again He would die, and again, and so for ever, by His own will rendered powerless against the free and evil wills of men.

Then Aske met the full assault of darkness without reprieve of hoped for light, for God ultimately vanquished was no God at all. But yet, though God was not God, as the head of the dumb worm turns, so his spirit turned, blindly, gropingly, hopelessly loyal, towards that good, that holy, that merciful, which though not God, though vanquished, was still the last dear love of a vanquished and tortured man . . .

By this time that which dangled from the top of the Keep at York, moving only as the wind swung it, knew neither day nor night, nor that it had been Robert Aske, nor even that it had been a man.

Even now, however, it was not quite insentient. Drowning yet never drowned, far below the levels of daylight consciousness, it suffered. There was darkness and noise, noise intolerably vast or unendurably near, drilling inward as a screw bites and turns, and the screw was pain. Sometimes noise, pain, darkness and that blind thing that dangled were separate; sometimes they ran together and became one.

But in his dying, his consciousness moved on, beyond a point where any of us are ever entitled to knowledge. The visions of Julian of Norwich are put into the mouth of, and translated, by Malle, a serving woman.

"God 'a mercy!" Malle cried, "God 'a mercy! Here He comes between the graves, out of the grave.

"When He was born a man," she said, "He put on the leaden shroud that's man's dying body. And on the cross it bore Him, bore Him down, sore heavy, blinding Him to the blindness of a man. But there, darkened within that shroud of mortal lead, beyond the furthest edge of hope, God had courage to trust yet in hopeless, helpless things, in gentle mercy, holiness, love crucified.

"And that courage, Wat, it was too rare and keen and quick a thing for sullen lead to prison, but instead it broke through, thinning lead, fining it to purest shining glass, to be a lamp for God to burn in.

"So men may have courage," she said . . .

But Robert Aske had gone too far, nor did he need now that Malle should tell him.

For now (yet with no greater fissure between then and now than as a man's eyes are aware, where no star was, of the first star of night), now he was aware of One – vanquished God, Saviour who could as little save others as Himself.

But now, beside Him and beyond was nothing, and He was silence and light.

*

The centre of this pain, and also of this silence and light, lies in the Eucharist. Sometimes we are ill-served by familiarity. Even the language of the original events that we re-enact, Eucharist by Eucharist, has become so familiar to us that it has lost some of its force, partly through constant repetition. From the phraseology of picking up our cross, and following our Lord, we have to strip all the clothing of habit, take it back to its original meaning, and think of His torture and of His death on a gibbet. Sometimes I cannot understand our external placidity, as we stand there, faced now, afresh, with the agony of this death, and the flies on these wounds. The re-enactment is a burning-glass, focusing pain, drawing together all those screams I have heard, all those broken branches and bruised flowers, all those fossils in the Grand Canyon, all the fears I have for my own future of cumulative fracture. There is nothing, ultimately, nothing, that I can do of myself to transform all this pain. There have been times I have wanted to scream: times when yet another new bit of Bridget's body has given up, and I have not been able to bear to go at all. I do remember how once my own pain was transformed for me by pure gift, by the presence of the Crucified. Can I, like Robert Aske, depend upon that presence? All E can do is to offer the pain. sometimes the complete and stark accuracy with which the Eucharist embodies the totality of experience as I know it is in itself nearly unendurable. Like all total accuracy, it also brings relief. Then the Offertory is taken onwards, the action moves from Crucifixion to Resurrection. Easter is less comprehensible than good Friday, but I can at least, in the face of this silence and this glory, understand why Peter was reduced to chattering meaninglessly of building booths at the Transfiguration. Joy has to be silent. Or the only words are the Sanctus.

But it is because the celebration of the Eucharist and Christ's offering of Himself in it seems to comprehend all the realities of acute pain and death that I have not handed in my ticket. I have spoken openly here of suffering and of death, breaking my own taboos, because it seems to me that a faith which cannot comprehend these realities, and contain them within its central paradox of life through God's death, is not worth having. We have to learn to live in the tension which seems so much the crux of Christianity, in which present agony is also permeated with joy or the promise of joy. If we cannot, we are only subscribing to pious platitudes. So our own discovery that events which stretch us to the limit, and then beyond what we think we are capable of, these times of acute suffering can bring with them an insight into joy beyond our rational conception, is fundamental to our growth. I can at least bear witness to some of this kind of reality.

*

I do not remember when I started to pray. Where do the roots of a craving for God come from? Like all growth, with me, it was slow. There were no lights on the road to Damascus. I was fortunate in many ways to have had no religious teaching from my benevolent agnostic parents: there was nothing to need to lose. The Primitive Methodist rediscovered in my mother after her stroke did not appeal to me. The nearest I ever came to the Damascus road sort of experience was typically low-key. One day when I was working on manuscripts in the University Library in Cambridge, I was bored by the type of document I was reading. I had got my searching time, for the kind of evidence I was looking for, down to two minutes per folio. I was suddenly distracted by the utterly irrelevant thought that the four most dynamic people I knew, the four most filled with life, and the four least shockable people, to whom you could tell anything, all had something in common. They crossed the Church spectrum from Roman Catholic to Quaker, but they were all practising. In no other respect did they share anything. "Odd", I thought. Like Clement Attlee considering the effects of the atomic bomb, I said, "I must look into that". Then I looked at the clock in the Manuscript Room. I had wasted, or spent, twenty minutes, ten folios of precious time.

The first landmark had happened long before. It was the Eucharist, which first disclosed some utterly unforeseen, unexpected intimations of glory to me. I suppose there must have been some external indication that this was going to be important, for I was given Thomas Merton's *Elected Silence* for a confirmation present. I began to wonder about contemplative prayer. For my twenty-first birthday, a perceptive friend gave me the Lady Julian's *Revelations of Divine Love*, and the covers became worn. But my wonderings did not take me very far: when I eventually arrived at what became my abbey, fifteen or so years later, the Abbess asked me why I had taken so long to get there. "Were you frightened of nuns?" she asked. "No," I answered, "I am a historian. I was frightened of God." She seemed to understand perfectly.

My abbey has been very important to me. The density and opaqueness of contemplative silence is impossible to convey: in it there is room for movement and life of unexpected kinds. I never know what I go there for: the meaning comes out in the silence, and has never, so far, been one I knew of in advance. Of all the psalms, the eighty-fourth expresses it most accurately:

> How lovely is your dwelling place,
> O Lord of hosts.
> My soul longs, yes, faints,
> for the courts of the Lord,
> my heart and flesh sing for joy to the living God.

Despite, or because of, the sheer brutal hard work of presenting all the hard truths in my life to be transformed, and the terrifying meaning and all-inclusiveness of the post-communion prayer "Here we offer and present to you, O Lord, ourselves, our souls and bodies, to be a reasonable, holy, living sacrifice", my oblation there is fundamental to me. I find a depth of joy there that I do not often know elsewhere. It is for some reason easy for me to look at God and love Him: at my abbey, very, very easy. But although it has been made easy for me to look at Him, and I have loved Him for a long time, so long is the road to perfection in love, that only sometimes, very recently, have I begun to know that He looks back at me with any love. I need to learn much more.

I cannot remember when I started to pray the *Sanctus*. I do not know whether all those hospital clinics, at which it never seemed possible to work academically, all those gifts of unplanned time I resented so bitterly to start with, actually formed the habit. Or perhaps the habit transformed them. I do a lot of waiting, anyway: people who are not infrequently immobilized, or who have to rest a lot, do. I was aided perhaps by the view from my window. For seventeen years, our bedroom looked out westwards into the trees of an eighteenth-century park. The form and structure of those trees, and the clear gold light that outlined them, meant a very great deal to me. I am tempted to say what is palpably untrue, that only the housebound really learn to appreciate landscape. "The world is charged with the grandeur of God." In some bad times, I lived on the shadow-tracery of leaves, reflected on my wall. At some point, my mind and attention began to be taught to use these periods of waiting to try to pray. At some point, I must have been grasped by some perception of the beauty of God. So my mind started to slip into the words of the *Sanctus* when it was not otherwise engaged, as, of course, it usually was, and is. I tried once to change this accustomed background mutter of "Holy, holy, holy", into the words of the Jesus prayer, which seemed to be recommended. But it did not work, so I stopped trying. At some later point, I discovered St Teresa of Avila's *Way of Perfection*. I have still not got beyond the introductory chapters, and doubt whether I ever will. There seems no point in reading beyond what I can understand. However I do not comprehend how people can write, as one author I read recently did, "There are times when the sort of prayer God gives us is the rather empty experience known as the prayer of quiet". If this experience is empty, I cannot imagine riches.

There is a completeness about attentive silence in the presence of God that leaves nothing else for me to desire. I am ashamed that so often idleness or busyness and a lack of sense of priorities squeeze out the time in which I could at least put myself in the way of achieving this stillness. I cannot imagine why I am not better organized, since on the rare occasions when I am, all that I most desire is sometimes given to me, and I seem completed. The only problem is that there *is* a completeness about adoration: the soul is stilled in the presence of God, there is nothing left to desire. Yet, given the limits of perception, and awareness, and the defect of will, attention quivers to a halt. One has to come back. Why then do I not make every effort to be there, the place where I most belong? Why am I so invincibly idle, and so negligent?

*

God has a black sense of humour. By the time I discovered that I had a strong drive towards the contemplative, I had been happily married for years, and was extremely busy. Increasingly, however, as time goes on, vocations fuse, and a strict distinction between life as a secular, and life as a religious, seems inapplicable to me.

The acceptance of limitation seems to me one of the most important, and also one of the most dangerous, of disciplines. If you live in a prison cell, it is foolish to spend energy beating yourself into a pulp against the walls: but before accepting those walls, you have to make sure they are there, and that you have made every effort to escape from them. Only the inescapable should be accepted. Everything that can be amended, transformed, healed, or ameliorated has to be done first. Teilhard de Chardin wrote:

> At the first approach of the diminishments, we cannot hope to find God except by loathing what is coming upon us and doing our best to avoid it. The more we repel suffering at that moment, with our whole heart and our whole strength, the more closely we cleave to the heart and action of God.[12]

12 Pierre Teilhard de Chardin, *On Suffering* (Collins, London, 1975), trs. from *Sur La Souffrance*, (Editions du Seuil, 1974) p.69. H.A. Williams has also written splendidly on establishing whether necessity is truly so, and then, *if* it is, making it the medium of creativity in *Tensions* (Mitchell Beazley, London 1976, pp. 104-6, and Fount Paperbacks, 1988).

My own prison cell, since the disease stabilized as I was promised, is the kind of low-grade grinding discomfort that my somewhat battered spine presents me with. One of the worst positions, unfortunately for me, is sitting writing, as my craft demands. So my life is lived in a series of short bursts. I alternate sitting and lying: I live in a series of two- or three-hour stretches. The pain is not bad at all: but there is something exhausting about the monotonous way it goes on, and on, and on. There is no thermometer for pain, but I have found it is often a bit worse than that of a broken rib. I am very thankful for the pain-killers on which I live, but they only blur it. I cannot imagine what it would be like to be really comfortable in one's body. If I neglect the ache for too long, it mounts to a level that distracts me from any sort of coherent thought.

There is a further complication that if I ignore the discomfort for too long, it can also lead to muscular spasm, which bends me double, and can put me to bed in a relatively helpless state, which is tiresome for me, and more so for my family. This has been a peculiarly difficult manifestation: it is not a recognized side-effect of the disease at all, and worried me lest I should be attempting to escape some of the undoubted complications of my life, by going to bed, however uncomfortably. My own old adolescent fears of psychosomatic illness came to the fore. Psychiatric assessment, which seemed very necessary, to make sure that I was not sub-consciously seeking extra and unnecessary limitation, did not give any insight at all, this time. Much more insight was given by an observant GP, who noticed that these attacks of muscular spasm only assaulted me in the second half of the month, and were relieved as if by magic at the end of it. Older women who develop osteoporosis do not observe in themselves these phases of the moon. There was also a question of whether my lost battles with the bed and the washing-machine had left their marks on my person, in residual small mechanical damage. Moreover, while some of the worst and most strenuous episodes of caring for our

91

daughter did not coincide with muscular spasm, it succeeded quite frequently in preventing me from doing things I loved. It seemed that it, too, was to be accepted as a physical limitation, rather than as an avoidance technique, and I must get on with using the times of isolation and relative immobility it gave me as profitably as possible. So I have come to a working arrangement, which is the best I can achieve.

When the discomfort has become so great that I can do nothing but lie down, and cannot think clearly, then I know my work has become prayer. While I am still sitting at my desk, I am still a historian. The confusing bit is the bit in between, when I am not sure whether I am still trying to think, or have become so uncomfortable that it is time to try to pray. This does seem a very churlish way to treat God: to attempt to focus on Him only when my attention is distracted by the discomfort is curiously unceremonious. His humility appears endless. However, the humility of other historians is not to be relied on in the same way. But using the apparently unavoidable pain as profitably as possible means continuing to do academic work "upside down" as much as I can, and attempting to be aware of the presence of God.

It is very good to have something to try to do with the pain. While it still remains an unmitigated evil, I can yet regard it somehow as a means to an end. I cannot describe the process very well, but I have found it to be one of somehow *absorbing darkness* – a physical or mental suffering of my own, or worse, of someone else's – into my own person, my own body, or my own emotions. We have to allow ourselves to be open to pain. Yet all the while we must resist any temptation to assent to it being other than evil. If we are able to do this, to act, as it were, as blotting-paper for pain, without handing it on in the form of bitterness or resentment or of hurt to others – then somehow in some incomprehensible miracle of grace, some at least of the darkness may be turned to light. It can also be used as a reminder to focus on what is really important. Unlike impending execution, it does not concentrate the mind wonderfully; indeed, pain scatters concentration for the most part. But its emphatic attack on the body, its almost annihilating powers, can be made helpful if they serve to scatter what is inessential in our feeling. Teilhard wrote, "God has already transfigured our sufferings by making them serve our conscious fulfilment. In his hands, the forces of diminishment have become perceptively the tool that cuts, carves and polishes within us the stone".[13] It may be tempting, in chronic pain, to give up on the body, to despair of it; but the Word was made flesh. It seemed, and seems, important to me that the incarnate Christ came to us, and into our world of ramshackle bodies. Mine is so very ramshackle that sometimes it is difficult to be patient with it, but I do try. I enjoy material things a lot, which helps. It is only the *wrongness* I object to. I loathe and detest my bone disease. I am often miserable, often shamefully discontented, often isolated, often lonely. I fear pain, and the fear does not grow less. But oddly, after twenty years, I can no longer wish that things were quite otherwise, except for my husband's sake. Learning to live with the disorder as creatively as possible has in the end formed the person I am. I cannot, in the last resort, regret being the person I am, as historian, or mother, or oblate. I think I can say, without any trace of masochism, that the disease has indeed been a creative medium. I have tried to use the pain of it to remind me to try to focus on what is really important. And what is really important is adoration.

13 Teilhard de Chardin, *op. cit.*, p.78

# SEVEN

*∽∿∽∿∽∿∽∿∽∿∽∿∽∿∽∿∽∿∽∿∽∿∽∿∽*

## *Bridget, II*

No worst, there is none. Pitched past pitch of grief,
More pangs will, schooled at forepangs, wilder wring.
Comforter, where, where is your comforting? . . .
O the mind, mind has mountains; cliffs of fall
Frightful, sheer, no-man-fathomed. Hold them cheap
May who ne'er hung there.

GERARD MANLEY HOPKINS[1]

While I was learning my craft as a historian, and beginning
to learn to pray, Bridget was moving on. The gerbils of her
infancy were succeeded by terrapins, which did not make
such inroads into fabric; also by a bad kitten, which, when it
arrived, had its paws dipped in finger-paint to make Bridget's
Christmas card. It grew big enough to distinguish itself by
stealing a whole leg of lamb, marinaded with garlic, from the
Professor of Sociology, who lived next door. The play-group
was succeeded by infant school. My minute daughter and I
distinguished ourselves one day by staggering in with what,
in the far distance, we had taken to be a "twig" suitable for
the autumn "nature table" in the reception class: it took three
teachers to shift it sensibly, and it eventually occupied an
outsize bucket in the corner of the large school hall for
Assembly.

That infants' school was the best in the area, and the staff

---

1 "No worst, there is none", *Poems by Gerard Manley Hopkins*, ed.
Norman H. Mackenzie (Folio, London 1974) p.112

were splendid. It was not altogether easy for them, though. By the time Bridget was four, she had learned to drink all her fluids, and all her medicine, even the potassium chloride, which is sufficiently potent to blister, and then strip, paint, if you knock over the medicine glass. Whatever was predictable in her care had been made as routine, and unobtrusive, a matter as possible: the Secretary of the History Department kept a stencil and ran off batches of sheets of foolscap fluid charts as we filled them up, day after day, after day. But the work of filling them up *right* still had to be done. Primary school staff, however good, cannot really be asked to keep track of a twenty-four hour fluid chart, and make sure it comes out right: nor can they administer more than a strictly limited number of glasses of medicine. She was very frequently sick in class, too, because kidney failure manifests itself that way. Oddly, I seemed to have less working time once she started school, because I was more frequently on the road, when I was myself mobile, in and out, collecting her to sort out the chart and the medicines and taking her back again. The other children were kind, and accepted her. But the playground was impossible for her: she was half the size of the others, and still very fragile.

The headmistress was such a remarkable woman that she joined the other, rare, figures in my private pantheon. I cannot remember which of Bridget's particular admissions to hospital caused her to summon me. She was concerned about our son, higher up her school. "Look," she said, "you all try to be super-human all the time: you all pretend all this weight of nursing responsibility you carry, and your own illness, is entirely normal. It is not. It is confusing for the child: he needs to *know* that sometimes his father worries, and sometimes his mother cries." It was interesting advice. I do not remember that we took it: but I did start to think about laughter.

The habit of laughter does serve a genuine purpose, which often liberates. I remember the occasion when I had broken my right wrist, and my left leg. Perhaps a gymnast could have managed mobility on crutches, but I could not. The student who meant so much came to live with us for a fortnight, so that my husband could fulfil the obligations of an honorific Visiting Professorship abroad. In that fortnight, inevitably, an ophthalmic appointment we had been waiting for for months came up for Bridget at the Hospital for Sick Children. We were deeply worried about her eyesight: it seemed essential I should go to hear what the new specialist said. Our GP laid on the necessary ambulance transport to put me on to, and take me off, trains. The attendant girl came too, to help. After the appointment I was tired, there was a gap between trains, and I asked, stupidly in a children's hospital, if I could lie down somewhere. Of course, there were only cots. "There are examination couches in Outpatients," said a helpful nurse, "perhaps those would be long enough?" She wheeled me down. When I stood up in the examination cubicle on my one good leg, the bed was well above hip-height. "Well, you could just *stand* on this chair," said the helpful nurse, "and then climb on to the bed." It was no good: I doubled up with quite genuine helpless laughter at the impossibility of the request. The nurse looked alarmed. "Don't worry," said the girl with me, who knew me very well, "when she's finished laughing, she'll just stand on that chair, like you said . . ."

I think laughter at your own utter absurdity brings home your own total inadequacy and dependence on grace, which is very necessary, considering the mammoth efforts situations like that require you to make. A strong sense of the absurd is a very useful ally.

But laughter can also accidentally turn into armour-plating, and imprison the wearer. Sometimes grief does need expression. We had so much stress to carry that we were desperately afraid of boring anyone with it. It is perhaps from me that Bridget has caught the extremely bad habit of saying everything is "fine", even to those who really need, or want, to know, when it is not. The people we came, rightly, to value most highly were those with whom we could be honest, and those from whom we did not feel we had to shield our grief or anxiety. They were very rare indeed; such grown-ups are: but our daughter's godparents, mercifully, were of that kind.

When she came to the top of the infant school, we were summoned again by the headmistress. She did not honestly feel Bridget could proceed normally into the junior school: the problems with the playground, fluid chart, and the constant sickness were too great. I was devastated: we had fought so hard for normality, and here was a definition of failure. The headmaster of the special school for physically-handicapped and delicate children, which then still existed in our local area, was obviously accustomed to this reaction when he saw us. I was astonished, however, that he apparently intended to be responsible for her during the entire school day. It took a long time to explain the mechanics of medicine, and fluids, and care: he did not turn a hair. Years later, he told me she was the most complex child medically they had ever had to look after, and they were not quite sure they could manage. At the time, you would not have known he felt there was any problem. Here was another figure for my pantheon.

After she moved, we gradually watched another transformation in her. Despite the excellence of her infant school, she had stood out as "different". No group of six-year-olds are really good at having one of their number constantly being sick in lessons. We lived in what was defined then as a "backward" paediatric area. What this meant in practice was that the children with cystic fibrosis, with heart murmurs from rheumatic fever, and bad asthma, went to the special school, along with the victims of spina bifida and cerebral palsy. They were all normally intelligent; "slow learners" went to another unit. In this group of children, everyone had a physical problem. Bridget was at last quite "ordinary" and normal. This was new. What was more, the staff were not afraid. When she was well, they pushed her quite hard intellectually, an exercise she thoroughly enjoyed. When she was unwell, she slept on a mattress in the corner of her classroom, and they looked after her. They never got it wrong. She blossomed. I am really not at all sure about the recommendations of the Warnock Report. It is so important, we learned from that experience, for a child to be ordinary: in this special school, our daughter could be just that. As for me, I was liberated. It was the first time since she was born that I was not responsible for her care, during school hours at least, and I could actually get on with my own work in complete freedom, knowing she was both cared for, and happy. It was wonderful. Although my skills as a historian had not deteriorated over the previous, splintered years, it was quite a different experience to be able to exercise them spaciously, as it were.

I do not remember when she and I developed the vulgar habit of swearing solidarity on the way to a hospital admission by spitting on our palms, and shaking hands. It was a good pledge, and sometimes, in a tight corner, we still use it. It conveys more reassurance than realms of words could. Outside her periods in hospital, I could now get on with my own life: when she was in, she needed me.

We had been warned she would die between seven and fourteen. She was only eight when the consultant at Great Ormond Street said he had now enough points on his graph to be sure she only had another six months or so to live. That afternoon, I borrowed a push-chair, and took her to the Zoo. The habit of normality was strongly laid on us: it was raining, so we were extravagant, and bought extra tickets for the shelter of the Aquarium. To this day, I can see the great white-plated bellies of turtles as they swim upwards in their tank in front of me, up to, and over, my head height. It had been all very well knowing intellectually that she would die: now the reality was on me. Next, we watched the archer-fish, who catch their prey above the water by shooting it down with globules of spit. It was a good afternoon, and she enjoyed it.

*

It is no one's fault that both she, and I, live, and have lived all this time, "on the frontiers of medical knowledge", although I do sometimes wish they would find a fresh phrase for it. When she was one, we had been told kidney transplants were irrelevant in this disease. We had learned to live with what we had been told was the accurate foreknowledge of her death. Now we were told that transplants in the States had shown that the incoming kidney was not after all affected by the disease, although no one then understood why not. A transplant could be tried, if we wanted, and we could perhaps, if there was no rejection, adjust ourselves to the prospect of her life.

That first time we were offered a transplant when she was eight, the success rate was only fifty per cent after two years. It is now much higher. They left us to find out for ourselves that the success rate for donor kidneys was as high as eighty per cent, since the Hospital for Sick Children was very scrupulous not to indulge in anything which could feel like emotional blackmail. She felt so very normal, that on these figures, the offer of a parental kidney felt appropriate. We then got transferred to the transplant unit at Guy's. It is always hard to lose paediatricians you know and trust, because you have worked together for so long. It was much more distressing for me when my husband turned out to be the more suitable donor: I badly wanted one of us to be kept intact and viable, and my very inept body seemed so much more suitable as a source for spare parts.

The whole procedure was then so experimental, that they left it as late as possible, so that she was sleeping practically all the time. That summer we discovered the island of Iona, and she lay sleeping on the white sand by the sea for most of our holiday before the admission. By then, she needed a fortnight's dialysis before the transplant, so that the new kidney did not face an impossible chore cleaning up the sewage in her bloodstream. Fitting the plastic tubing to artery and vein in her calf, so that she could be attached to a machine, was not pleasant. The many scars from the many cut-downs of her infancy were now joined by new and bigger ones. I was afraid her nerve would crack before the transplant itself. Instead, she made a ridiculous fuss about a wobbly tooth she had. After a fortnight of that, I stupidly said, "Really, anyone would think you'd never had a wobbly tooth before!" She looked at me coldly, and said witheringly, "Would you rather I was complaining about other things?" She had always had a disconcerting gift of sudden insight, combined with blunt shrewdness. A few days after the transplant, when she was both properly round from anaesthetic, and at least reasonably comfortable, she looked at the library of favourite books I had packed, either to read to her or for her to read. "We got this all wrong," she said. "I don't count as eight at all, only six if that. *None* of this is any good."

That fortnight, and indeed the next week or two, was tough. In some ways I was most worried about our son. At eleven it is a lot to have one's sister perhaps dying, and one's father, however briefly, at risk on the same day. The new paediatric team was amazingly understanding when I said I wanted him on the ward with me during the actual kidney transplant. In my judgement, a highly intelligent and sensitive eleven-year-old was going to survive that sort of day better, if he could see what was happening, rather than do his own imagining, alone in a vacuum. Guy's said "Yes" without externally turning a hair. The last thing anyone can actually want in an intensive care cubicle is an inquisitive eleven-year-old asking how the machinery works, particularly during a procedure which was then still fairly experimental. But they still allowed it. It helped me carry my elder normal child through the transplant quite enormously.

As for me – bizarrely, and, like all such developments, quite unplanned – I started to discover some reality in a bit of the doctrine of the Church that had previously been quite irrelevant. I walked around, those weeks, feeling as if I was imprisoned behind a very thick plate-glass wall. People were immensely kind: they mouthed words through the glass, just like fish, and just as meaningless. I responded, politely I hope, feeling totally unreal. My research supervisor, a short-tempered and deeply humane man with a gift of words, whom I had loved, had died some years before. Such was his care for me that he had come all the way to Great Ormond Street weekly for six months while Bridget was first in, to take me out to lunch to make sure I had a proper meal once a week. For five and a half of those months, he had never even mentioned his great love, Anglo-Saxon charters, to me. Quite correctly he gauged that I was unable to focus on scholarship. Now quite suddenly, inside the glass walls that cut me off from everyone, however kind, his presence was lent to me. It was utterly ordinary and familiar, as pithy-tempered, as ready to keep me up to the mark, and as kind, as ever. It was a very odd experience, and his company was withdrawn before the glass walls melted. But I felt that the Communion of Saints was a real concept, in a way that it had not been before.

*

Curiously enough, it is the high points of those years that stand out for me. When Bridget was only three, I had distinguished myself by going down with double viral pneumonia as the trees flamed into glory in October. That time, I lost my fight to stay out of the local hospital, being slow to take in that "illness" was different from bone-disease, which leaves you functioning. I began to understand when I failed to measure out 20mls of potassium for her, because my temperature was over 104, and I couldn't see straight, or think clearly. But the habit of trying to be there to give stability was too strong. My GP wanted to put me in. I refused. "You are breathing on a quarter of a lung: I'll give you twenty-four hours", he said. Twelve hours later, he came back. "You are breathing on only an eighth of a lung", he said. "I'm sorry, but if you are like this in the morning, I'm putting you in." "No!" I said. But in the morning, I lost. "Well, if you *want* to make it an emergency", he said ... As I slipped away into the benign fog, astonishingly I first lost my anxiety for my children. Then I lost my anxiety for my husband. When, some days later, I came back again out of my fog, it was to find an unknown night Sister standing by my bed. "I've been waiting to ask you," she said, "are you the mother of that baby that used to run the children's ward?"

After my month in hospital, I further distinguished myself, and eventually enraged our good and patient GP, by going down with pleurisy three times. Something had to be done. We decided to spend my small inheritance from my mother on going to Greece. My husband travelled with a helpful six-year-old son, a wife who fell over with weakness from time to time, a three-year-old daughter and her fluid chart, a crate of dextrose, another crate of medicines, and a drip machine, just in case he needed it. To start with, I simply slept in a bed he put in a grove of orange trees at the back of the cottage. I can smell them yet. But then I got better. We celebrated our daughter's fourth birthday, and our son's seventh, with picnics in the Hall of the Kings at Mycenae. You really can do extraordinary things, given determination.

Two years after the first kidney transplant, we travelled across Europe in the smallest size of Fiat van that will sleep four people, doing the field work for my husband's study of medieval trade routes, and using a fifteenth-century itinerary as a guide. The children were ten and thirteen. It was cold and had rained so much that the whole of North Europe was like a sponge. We were very happy. We discovered two universals: camp-sites were the same, wherever we were, unless the water in the showers was warm, which was very unlikely. And so was the Mass, whether in Flemish, French, Italian, or later, Czech. For the next three months Bridget and I did the marketing together in a little Italian hill town. She was, of course, much faster at picking up the language than I was. The odd thing about it was that we had planned the trip pre-transplant, and had intended to travel with the dextrose crate, the sterilizing and mixing equipment, and run the fluid chart. Given my husband's practical genius, I expect we would have done it. Instead, we merely had bottles of immuno-suppressants and insulin, under the seat, and blood tests to organize. But, as we discovered, after the children had had their eleventh and fourteenth birthdays in the Tuscan hills, eleven is about the top of the age-range you can make happy in a family environment, by family endeavour. After that, the need for a social group gets much bigger, and the limitation of parents as providers becomes more acute.

*

Bridget had developed diabetes. Neither she, nor I, was very "good" about that. We thought we had had enough, and we did not want to learn to live with another sort of a disease, however controllable. We were angry. The days of her wonderful special school were over, and so was my freedom from responsibility. I had one of her secondary school headmistresses on the telephone, asking me to be sure not to move out of reach of the instrument during all school hours. Bridget also met stupidity and incomprehension in her class-mates for the first time. For a year, she was sent to Coventry. Despite all this, quite remarkably she kept up with her peer group academically, as far as and including "O" levels. Her determination has always been extraordinary, as the night Sister I met somewhat unexpectedly when I had pneumonia, had observed. Taking her "O" levels involved coming out of hospital, where she was recovering after a hypoglaecaemic attack, in order not to miss the biology paper for which she had done all the revision. She still had double vision. Fortunately, the drawing section of the paper, which she had been dreading for months, only demanded a cross-section of a banana. She passed.

But after she had done a year in the sixth form, the world began to fall apart. To start with it had seemed quite suitable for her to begin on three "A" levels, but she missed most of the first half of the second year in a switch of immuno-suppressants, which involved going to clinics in London three times a week. She tried desperately to keep up, translating Catullus in the clinic corridors, but it did not, and could not, work. That was the first time her morale showed signs of cracking. Then, a year later, first she was diagnosed as partially sighted, and then almost immediately she went into renal failure again. We were taken utterly, and totally, by surprise.

*

When we had opted for a transplant, we were told the first two years were the crucial period, or perhaps the only period for which they had enough figures to be statistically reliable. Anyway, we were told the longer it went, the safer it was. We had agreed only on condition that if it failed, nobody would ask us to try a second transplant. When we got to the end of that two years, we enquired again, and were told there were new figures for five years post-transplant. "It seems", said the consultant, "if you get as far as eight years, you can probably forget to worry. The kidney is there for good." So when we got to eight years, we did stop worrying. We naturally did not enquire whether their knowledge had moved on again. They, equally naturally, did not volunteer information. So when she went into renal failure again after ten years, it was a complete shock to us. "Oh!" they said, in astonishment. "Didn't you know we have found out that transplanted kidneys go through an ageing process, and wear out?" "No", we said.

This kind of confusion is utterly unavoidable in a fast-moving new field, I think. It would have been utterly improper for us not to trust what we were told by the most advanced experts in the business: it would have been redundant for us to fret, and to ask useless extra questions. Our job in life was to keep our family happy and together, and after that to keep abreast of *historical* research, not try to keep informed about the state of medicine. This seemed to be an entirely necessary part of the discipline of living in the present moment. But the sort of intellectual and emotional adjustment you go through each time new information reaches you, and you have to reorganize your entire lives accordingly, is very great. Perhaps it would have been a little, but not much, more comfortable, if we had not had similar adjustments to make about the treatment of bone diseases at approximately the same time. For I was also going to those other clinics, and having bone-biopsies, in my spare time. Now we were faced with heart-searching, and conscience-searching of the most agonizing kind I have yet experienced. I had spent a large part of seventeen years of my life, and much of my maturity as an adult, in working quite hard and continuously to sustain our daughter, and enable her to be launched as a fully viable human being, in spite of what seemed almost impossible odds. My emotional and physical investment must be at least as high as that of the doctors involved. All medical instinct and training is to save life, to redeem, to try to heal. In this, paediatricians are at one with, and sometimes use, and trade on, the huge biological fund of parental instincts that will attempt most things if they are humanly possible.

Three times, because of these loving parental instincts, my husband and I had interfered with our daughter's attempt to die. In my pregnancy, she tried to abort, and we prevented it, as we so badly wanted another child. When she was dying in a provincial hospital aged one, I took her to London, where she was not allowed to die. Despite my fear that we could not bring her up normally able to trust and to love, by the grace of God, and a great deal of hard work (which things often go together, in my experience), parts of her childhood have been viable, with moments of great joy. The third time we saved her life, when together, parents and paediatricians in full consultation, my husband gave her a kidney when she was eight, was relatively free from emotional stress, because she seemed so normal, apart from kidney failure. The decision was not very difficult: although the living out of it was very costly. But the fourth time, when she went in to renal failure again at eighteen, we jibbed. Cystinosis is not a renal disease. We were told initially it would kill by renal failure "in the first instance". Kidney transplants for cystinotics are only a kind of very highly-sophisticated tinkering with symptoms. We had learned over time, as the doctors had learned from observing her and other cystinotics, that there was, in fact, quite a lot of "second instance". By now, she was diabetic, either because her pancreas was affected by the cystine, or because her liver, or muscles, could not absorb insulin on account of it. Her thyroid had been atrophied. She had lax ligaments, and her knee joints were affected; possibly, though no one knows, by the cystine. She had a malformed hip. She could not walk very far without pain. Her feet swelled so badly, possibly because of all the cut-downs and scarring, that she frequently could not get her shoes on. At that stage, her photophobia was bad enough to make major roads impassable, safely, by her alone. She was partially-sighted. Above all, her late adolescence had made her friendless, and acutely lonely. The pain of watching a girl of acute intelligence and sensitivity cope with all this was very great, even though her courage, and eager humour, were commensurately high. We began to wonder whether her adulthood could be made as viable as her childhood was. And agonizingly, we were so much less able to help a girl who was eighteen, than we had been to help a baby and a small child. One can create a universe for a small handicapped child, involving it in play-groups, infant and junior schools, as it develops. One cannot create a universe for an adolescent, who has lost her peer-group from the innate effects of disease, and too much isolating medical experience. By definition, she needs such a group above all things. Your job as a parent has now become one you ought to have completed, and cannot. You ought not to be there any longer, and yet you still are, useless, but needed. The brief is impossible.

Also, shamefully, we were suffering from a sort of long-term tiredness I could not have foreseen. You are less resilient to conquer the next obstacle in your early fifties than in your early thirties. We had learned by now that there always is a next obstacle. Moreover, the fifteen years' grace, and relative stability of bone I had been promised, were now up. On the side, or in the background, we were facing that set of medical consultations too. Who was going to look after our daughter if I started to fracture? My husband had frequently performed the impossible, but looking after both of us, simultaneously, might be too much even for him. There was practically no provision for care for chronically-sick, young adults in the community, I had discovered,[2] especially if they were of normal, or high, intelligence, as she was. Anyway, to let her down was unthinkable, if she could not move on from home normally. We had never been able to find any kind of substitute care arrangements, and the days when a good au pair could solve some of our problems were long gone. There was even a selfish element that needed to be brought to the light, and faced, to see how much it was influencing our judgement: we wanted to be able to live our own professional lives, and travel, while I could still move.

All this would probably not have shaken us, if the next obstacle had not been the highest yet. Almost accidentally, we had heard that of the thirty or so young adult cystinotics in the world who had survived with the aid of kidney transplants, three had died of some form of neurological disease, "dementia" for short, until they invent a new medical term, that killed through brain damage by progressively destroying the functions of the nervous system, while leaving the young creature who suffered it fully conscious, sensate, aware.

There was no scientific proof that these cases were necessarily connected to the disease. They might have been the

2 John Harrison, *The Young Disabled Adult* (Report of the Royal College of Physicians, London 1986)

result of random chance. Moreover, there was a new drug, not yet through clinical trials, which for the first time tackled the root causes of the disease, rather than tinkering with the symptoms. It appeared to stop the deposit of cystine. The tune of the renal specialists changed from "We won't offer her another kidney", to "We'll just pop one in".

But I was slow to adjust, as always, to the existence of this new drug. I had been rocked back on my heels by the discovery of the dementia. Suddenly, I struck. The world came off its hinges.

No worst, there is none. Pitched past pitch of grief,
More pangs will, schooled at forepangs, wilder wring . . .

I had known since I was ten that the unimaginable worst could happen. If this dementia happened to our daughter, it felt like a definition of it. We seemed to be living in one of those insane, supremely logical, drawings by Esscher. They are mathematical, flawless, supremely logical, or rather you cannot perceive the flaw in the logic. You find yourself in them eventually walking up some staircase that cannot be there, over an abyss that has no bottom. They are the fabric of nightmare, which is drawn in another mode by Francis Bacon and Edvard Munch. This world of genuinely humane, high-technology, modern medicine in which we were living, suddenly felt like that. I could see she would now never be allowed to die of kidney failure, which I knew to be benign, if her last near-death was anything to go by, for they had let her almost sleep herself out when she was eight before they embarked upon anything so experimental as a transplant then was. Nor could she decide against another transplant herself, which would be tantamount to suicide, for she was such a triumphant person, and a fighter. She was alive because of her determination, anyway. Instead, because there was no logical reason why not, and these cases of "dementia" were not yet scientifically proven to be attached to cystinosis, she

108

would be encouraged onwards by her doctors. Perhaps, after all, she would develop it. If so, they, like us, would lament, for they genuinely cared for her. But then they would have their proof. Another scientific advance would have been made. They would have a scientific *reason* for not doing further transplants for cystinotics, unless, of course the new drug did prove effective. We were, after all, as we had been repeatedly told for years, on the frontiers of medical knowledge. But if the disease did, or could, in some cases, lead to "dementia", there was no reason to suppose prayer would stop it happening to this loved girl, when we had all interfered, yet again, to prevent a natural death. I could see no reason why we should blame the Almighty this time. Nor could we blame Him for the tribulations that had come on her since we prevented her death with the first transplant either. On the other hand, from the doctors' point of view, if the "dementia" did not happen, she would live. It was a risk they were willing to take for her in order to preserve her life. We were not.

Under the pressure of decision-making like that, the fabric of reason and order seemed all split from crown to base for me. The mind has mountains, cliffs of fall, and I was falling off them. One can understand those who would be mad, if only they could thereby abnegate thought. But the attempt to make right choices is not so lightly put aside: nor is madness, or irresponsibility, so lightly invoked.

*

The final twist was, however, that none of the decision-making was now ours. Finally, this fourth time, we had struck, at more medical interference. But she was now nineteen. Legally, the choice was nothing to do with us: indeed, it came as something of a shock to be told later that we would have been taken to the High Court if she had gone into renal failure again when she was only fifteen or sixteen, and we had not backed a further transplant, even before the advent of the new drug. When we embarked on all this, and I caught the London train when she was one, we did not know that it would be like being caught up in some vast machine. However, if the decision and the power were nothing to do with us, the responsibility of the background care was still entirely ours. Only legal and medical fiction could, and did, pretend otherwise. And to be utterly powerless, and almost completely responsible, is a bad combination.

But where was the girl, in all this? She had the brutal experience of choosing life for herself, not death, and knowing her parents would choose death. She did not know about the dementia, the knowledge that had finally swung us against further interference. The doctors did not tell her, or did not tell her in any form she could comprehend, and we could not, feeling she was too young for such a load, though not, it seemed, too young to be asked to choose life or death. So she chose, not knowing what she chose, or why we would have chosen otherwise. The depths of rejection were potentially immense. She, and we, were put in impossible positions.

We spent the next year, once she had chosen, swinging all our weight behind her, in the effort to make sure that she still knew she was loved. We were much helped, in a way I could have node without, and at a price she could have done without paying, when in a corridor she overheard one of the senior members of the hospital team instructing medical students on the possible effects of cystinosis. So she did get to know about the dementia. I wish she had not. She came raging home, and said, "Why didn't you *tell* me? You never *lied* to me before." Her fear was, and is, very great. her new adult consultant told her that he did not go around considering the statistical odds of having a heart attack, which applied to him, as this statistical risk applied in a like manner to her. He has been wonderful, both imaginative and down-to-earth. But still she lives with this impossible fear. "She cannot do other," he says, "she is too intelligent not to find out, or to overhear." He paid her the most massive compliment I have ever heard, quite accidentally, one that justified all the work of all the past. He told me of the way he used the letter of referral that came to him from the paediatricians to amaze visiting specialists to his clinic. Apparently it was unusual in its length, and in containing so many separate heads of different medical problems. "Their eyes glaze," he said, "and they expect her to be wheeled in on a stretcher with the drips up. They expect her to be an emotional and physical wreck. Then she bounces in, and cracks a joke, and their eyes nearly pop out of their heads." Her courage and resourcefulness are amazing. It is good to be able to admire one's own daughter.

*

The main piece of learning for me in that last kidney transplant was the necessary distancing of a child on the edge of adulthood with severe medical problems. Being an adult is choosing, and bearing, your own pain. Letting your child go free in an abnormal situation is not helping her to leave home, as you would both like, but choosing life rather than death at the price it costs. Letting your child go free is letting her choose the risk of dementia, unknowing. There was never such a purging of love. Yet withdrawing, as you should, you are still needed, not to protect her from the pain as you used to try, unavailingly, to do, but to put your arm around her when she panics at the top of that staircase, perceiving the abyss for herself.

I was useless at it, to start with. We were unfortunate that she had not been lengthily in hospital in her mid-teens, when I could have helped her learn to cope with the ward rounds herself, more suitably. Now she was admitted at the top end of the paediatric age-range, and she had never done this for herself before. We still spat into our palms, and shook hand in a tight spot. She begged me to be there, and so I still was, trying to teach her to her own spokeswoman as unobtrusively as I could. Letting her go free to assume her own pain, to stop trying to protect her, was difficult. I do not think I had ever been over-protective when she was out of hospital: I had wanted her to do things normally too much to try to avoid the inevitable attendant risks, and I had had too much deeply engaging work of my own to do to want to assume unnecessary maternity. But hospital, which must *seem* such a profoundly safe place to doctors, since all physical and nursing risks are covered, is different. To me "hospital" was the one place she could not safely be left, in case the scar-tissue that covered all those repeat experiences of her infancy which had terrified her so much, got ripped off again. I was chained to those memories, and that terrible year of her infancy. And I did not know that she was not, also.

So in hospital, even in her late teens, I stuck with her, just in case the old wounds did get re-opened, and also because she asked me to. I must have seemed grossly over-protective, for incomprehensible reasons, since these people were necessarily unaware of her past in any imaginative sense. They had thick files of notes in store, but that is different. I irritated the paediatricians, although they remained tolerant. Once old memory did re-open: someone in a hurry dug a piece of razor blade into her finger to do a blood-test.[3] I thought that I knew why she screamed. So once again I sat through investigations, kidney biopsies, the lot, just in case she should wake up and call "Mummy!" as she had so often before.

\*

Even if the lesson of the last few years has been that you must not and cannot protect your child from living, or from pain either, there is a profound irony. She still needs us available to give her a sense of security and of being continuously loved through these experiences, even though we are now totally powerless. We are, as it were "invisible" since she is an "adult". Yet we are still also completely responsible. And the years of grace and stability of bone I was promised have run out. Now she has failed, inevitably in all this medicine, to

3 See above p.51

112

keep up with her peer group, to move on from home after her "A" levels, into further training or a job, she is often alone at home, often unwell, often agonizingly lonely.

Partly the problem is practical. With small children, it is easy to arrange replacement care, even to run a fluid chart. With lonely unwell young adults, it is not nearly so possible to find a substitute, to meet a much less precise set of needs. I have not solved this. I try to arrange any sort of appropriate activity I can think of. The temptation for me is to try to solace her emptiness by being always available myself. Even if I am, though, I cannot really help. A girl this age needs much more than a parent. So, for the very first time, it is easy to throw away my own life, stop doing the very many things I have to do, and let her loneliness dominate me. I am in much more danger of failing to make appropriate claims for myself than I was when she was very little. The natural sequence of growing seems to be for the adolescent to move gradually away into independent living, to row out from the shore, further and further to the horizon, returning again and again to the shore after longer and longer journeys, always welcomed, until at last the horizon is passed, and the beach is no longer relevant, becoming only a familiar and loved environment to visit from islands of your own. This is what one wants, and welcomes, for one's child.

In the young adult's disappearance over the horizon, painful but entirely welcome, lies the beginning of a new sort of freedom for parents also. It is that we so much hoped for. We have so much to do together. It is quite different from this "normal" development to have a young adult at home, unable to move on. To carry on with your own life, you have in effect to go out and do your own work, knowing that behind you is a miserable vacuum. The awareness of the emptiness I leave behind in order to live my own life is always with me, like a convict's ball and chain. I cannot be free of it. Yet the situation seems to call for what feels like an unnatural remedy. Otherwise we might all be overwhelmed by handicap. I am helped, and humbled, by Bridget's own wisdom and generosity. She sent me away, for instance, to write this book, knowing that for her the time would be desolate.

*

We are profoundly thankful to have had this daughter, who has enriched us beyond belief, partly through pain I could not have dreamt of. She is, in herself, a triumph. Yet I have come seriously to doubt whether life should be sustained when it can only be done through massive and repeated medical intervention, especially when there is no community care, apart from the family, to which these young adults can suitably move on. Who is going to sustain the quality of this girl's life, when we physically no longer can?

Moreover I am no more inured to the pain of small children than I was at the beginning. A friend once said to me, "There are only two sorts of people, parents and non-parents". I do seriously doubt whether tiny children should be subjected to such prolonged emotional stress and inevitable scarring in the efforts to sustain their lives. I was told a story when Bridget was twenty. Its purpose was to illustrate how foolish I had been to resist a second kidney transplant. A baby had been born with a cleft lip and palate – not too agonizing at all. But in a short while it was observed that the baby also had a really exotic liver condition, so exotic that it was of interest even to the specialized liver unit. However, that was likely to clear up. The liver investigation showed some evidence of kidney malfunctioning, so the baby was passed on to the renal unit, where indeed it was found to need considerable help. By then it was also decidedly blue, so the paediatricians had a look at its heart. Extensive heart surgery was necessary, as kidney surgery would be too. While they looked at all this, they discovered a twisted gut. At that stage, my informant said, they had serious doubts. If there had been neurological evidence of any brain problem, they would not have started on the necessary lengthy programme of interference and redemption. But there was no such evidence, so they began. God alone knew how long this baby would be in hospital, or how many operations it would have, or how much pain and parental deprivation it would undergo. But *"There was no reason why not"*, said my informant. That doctor happened to be the consultant I most respected and trusted, who, like Bridget's Professor long before, thought of love as well as science. No wonder they saw no reason not to treat Bridget. In this world of advanced medicine, my husband and I are like some latter-day primitive Jehovah's Witnesses, resisting something as straightforward and life-saving as a blood transfusion would be.

But we still wonder even whether it is proper for a child to live from kidney transplant to kidney transplant, given that they are now known to wear out. The ethical problems are immense, and we are all surely feeling our way round a very grey area. Neither the response "Just pop in a kidney" nor ours "No child ought to be subjected to this degree of stress", can be right. Both are much too simple. If we adopt the paediatrician's approach, we may very well end up in a drawing by Esscher. Paediatricians never look at their results twenty years on. If we adopt our own approach, doctors might never have found out how to do something as life-saving and simple as an appendectomy.

There is no conclusion. I have no conclusion. We are all jointly engaged on redemptive work, which is, of its nature, agonizing. I would not, despite the agony, have missed it and the enrichment it has brought. But I do think it has taxed my husband and me almost to the limit, and there are times when I wonder frankly how much longer I can endure the pain and uncertainty of it. The situation itself is almost unendurable. Essentially, modern medicine sticks a family down on one of the "frontiers of medical knowledge" and says "Make your home here, and make it a good one; make your children secure, and safe, and loved". We try, but could anyone succeed?

# EIGHT

෴෴෴෴෴෴෴෴෴෴෴෴෴෴෴

# *Bones, II*

We must be still and still moving
Into another intensity
For a further union, a deeper communion
Through the dark cold and the empty desolation,
The wave cry, the wind cry, the vast waters
Of the petrel and the porpoise.
In my end is my beginning.

T.S. ELIOT[1]

This story has no end: or rather, I do not know its end. Here I am, in the still pool above the waterfall, going slowly round and round, waiting to see if the rapid acceleration of bone-loss I was warned of twenty years ago will happen to me this next year, or in the next three years, or not at all. I am being treated now with injections unknown twenty years ago, which may well arrest bone-loss. The immediate effects are very good, but in general their results are "statistically inconclusive", I am told. Twenty years is quite a long time, nearly half my conscious lifetime. For all that time I have "known" that I have had an active life until the menopause, and that then there was in front of me a cliff of fall of the unknown, or unfortunately not quite unknown, the gradual break-up of my skeleton while I still live in it. All knowledge, but not all fear, has for so long stopped there. I have worked

1 T.S. Eliot, "East Coker" (Faber and Faber, London) p.32

to live as fully as I could, knowing what might lie before me from the report of that coroner's inquest I read so long ago, and my own limited, but adequate, experience of acute pain when the children were little. That knowledge, that the known and possible would stop at a fairly precise point in time in front of me, was so complete, and I have so much tried to control my imagination about what lay beyond that, as a matter of discipline, that it has been very difficult to learn to hope at all. The idea of this new treatment is so relatively new to me, and still so inconclusive. Even the doctors are tentative: I do not think they have had many women who already have such thin bones going into the menopause, and as well as giving comfort and solace, as they do, they also feel scientific curiosity. So do I: I am, after all, the daughter of two scientists. But scientific curiosity does not allay terror. I fear to hope too much, as well. Supposing I do learn to hope for the postponement of the pain I dread so much, and am betrayed? Yet there is, I think, no record in the gospels of anyone coming to our Lord asking for healing and going away unhealed. Here am I, now being treated totally unexpectedly – since I was originally told there was no treatment – and apparently effectively. On the other hand, if He is the pattern for His followers, He spent a night in prayer in a garden. He prayed for the removal of agony, and, superficially, was not heard. Who am I to know what He wants of me? Is it at all possible that if I assent to living in my skeleton while it breaks up, if it does, He can be served by my pain? I still will not assent to the prospect of such pain as anything but a manifest evil. But St Paul wrote of filling up in his body the sufferings of Christ.[2] I am not St Paul, but I am part of the body of Christ. Do we, the whole Church, need to re-present in every generation, not only Christ's good news that we are loved, but also the suffering of Christ? Is this, in the end, the reasonable, holy and living sacrifice that might be asked? Such a vocation is terrifying,

2 Colossians 1:24-5

and I am incapable of it. But I have said that of the task in front of me so many times before. Only the alternative is worse, that such pain would be meaningless, a solitary exercise in agony. Pain is very anti-social, very isolating. So many people are too afraid of not knowing what to say, to dare to come near it. Am I compensating for this prospect of meaningless pain, by supposing it could in some way be used? I hope not, but self-deception is yet another pitfall.

This Juliantide, I have to renew my oblation as a Benedictine. This year we will begin to see whether my bones are eroding faster, or staying stable: this year they begin to be much at risk. So this Juliantide I have to be willing to do whatever is required of me, to go on with at least a semi-active life, to discover, after all, that the prognostications made twenty years ago were false, and to adjust joyfully to that, to write, and to teach and to travel, or to slide over the edge of my still pool into the roar of the water, and the pain. I cannot manage the perfect equipoise of hope, and the knowledge of the Garden. My mind will not contain both extremes. It is not big enough. All I have is the hardly prayable prayer of the Annunciation. I do not know what the will of God is for me: I know that in the gospels, disease was always healed by Him, wholeness was His will: but I also know of my own experience that pain, and fear, and dereliction can be assumed by Him. So either way is good. But how do I trust adequately to His mercy, shrinking as I am, and always have been, in the roar of the water, and the prospect of such possible pain? The sort of death Robert Aske died is conceivable for me, and I cannot endure it. It would mean dying truly beyond the limit of all faith, derelict and out of control, totally dependent on human opiates and on grace. I will have lost all sense of Him. Will He come? I do remember how acute pain was once transformed for me, by pure gift, by the presence of the Crucified. Can I, like Robert Aske swinging in his chains at York, ultimately depend on it?

This story has no end: or rather I do not know it. By the time I do, it will be too late to write it, and there will be no need any more. I shall make my oblation, and it will be hard, and all I will be able to say is "Be it unto me according to Thy word", the acceptance of either pattern, one of which is so much dreaded. So the constant redemption and making good of so much amiss continues, and I am full of joy allied with my own fear for the future. Whichever pattern is chosen for me, does not, in essence, matter, if either can also be redeemed. What does matter is that I should at last know myself, astonishingly, loved by God. If that monumental, extraordinary truth is so, then all manner of things will be well, at no superficial level, but at the end of the longest waterfall, even plummeting down the cliffs of fall within pain. For that realization, I depend on Him. Given it, in rare moments, I am possessed by joy. Whatever lies between me and it, the true end is written in a prayer of Bede,[3] that excellent historian and monk, who died dictating the end of a chapter, and whose last words, except for "Glory to the Father and the Son and to the Holy Ghost", were of his work: "It is well finished." He wrote in a prayer which survives:

We pray You good Jesus that as you have given us the grace to drink in with joy the Word that gives knowledge of you, so in your goodness you will grant us to come at length to yourself, the source of all wisdom, to stand before your face forever. Amen.

3  Bede, *A History of the English Church and People*, trs. and ed. Leo Sherley-Price (Penguin, Harmondsworth 1955) pp. 19-20

# NINE

# *The End*

Listen. The Word Himself calls to you to return, and with Him is the place of peace that shall not be broken, where your love will not be forsaken unless it first forsake. Things pass that other things may come in their place and this material universe be established in all its parts. "But do I depart anywhere?" says the Word of God. Fix your dwelling in Him, commit to God whatsoever you have: for it is from God. O my soul, wearied at last with emptiness, commit to Truth's keeping whatever Truth has given you, and you shall not lose any; and what is decayed in you shall be made clean, and what is sick shall be made well, and what is transient shall be reshaped and made new and established in you in firmness; and they shall not set you down where they themselves go, but shall stand and abide and you with them, before God who stands and abides forever.

Augustine, *Confessions*, IV, XI

O God of unchangeable power and eternal light,
look favourably on your whole Church, that
wonderful and sacred mystery; and by the tranquil
operation of perpetual providence carry out
the work of man's salvation; and let the whole
world feel and see that things which were cast
down are being raised up, and that things which
had grown old are being made new, and that all
things are returning to perfection through him from
whom they took their origin, even Jesus Christ our Lord.
AMEN.

Hide not Thy face from me. Let me see Thy face even if I die, lest I die with longing to see it.
The house of my soul is too small to receive Thee; let it be enlarged by Thee. It is all in ruins; do Thou repair it.

*Confessions*, I, V


Lord, Thy broken consort raise,
and the music shall be praise.

GEORGE HERBERT

Almighty God,
You have made us for yourself,
And our hearts are restless
Till they find their rest in you.
Teach us to offer ourselves to your service
That here we may have your peace,
And in the world to come may see you face to face;
Through Jesus Christ our Lord.
AMEN.

# Postscript

Two days after I returned home after writing this book, our daughter became ill with what was eventually diagnosed as the neurological failure described in Chapter 7. I have not substantially changed the text, and am happy to find I do not need, or wish, to do so. Her decline was in no sense amusing. However, she was given the gift of clarity and serenity in the last month of her life and was precisely aware of what was happening and to Whom she was going. It was a month which all four of us were mainly able to spend in her bedroom at home, reading aloud, listening to music, and surrounded by flowers.

She died in all our arms, very soon after her twenty-second birthday on the Sunday after Ascension Day, 1989.

This book was first published, strangely, a few days after her death. Before her death, I had already started work, with a group of concerned people, founding a hostel for severely disabled or chronically sick university students in Cambridge. When it was clear she was dying, these people suggested naming the hostel after her, and asked her permission to do so. She took great pleasure in it, for she felt she 'had done nothing'. This book, and Bridget's Hostel, are both quite unexpected and unlooked-for fruits of her life.

We have also set up 'Bridget's Trust' to help with the costs of caring for students with disabilities. Bridget herself wanted badly to go away from home to do a degree course, but nowhere she wanted to go could give her the nursing care she needed. A severely disabled student in the hostel is as expensive to look after as a patient in a 'cheap' hospital bed or even someone in prison. An endowment is therefore slowly being built up to secure the future of the hostel's caring work. We desperately need contributions, however small, to keep Bridget's Hostel in being (British gifts may be sent direct to the Treasurer, Bridget's Trust, Bridget's, Tennis Court road, Cambridge CB2 1QF, whilst North American gifts may be chanelled through the American Friends of Cambridge University, c/o The President, Stephen C. Price, Price and Zimmerman, 305 Harrison St SE, 3rd Floor, Leesburgh, VA 22075 (tel. 703-777-8850). The appropriate tax concessions naturally apply both in Britain and North America.)

I would be very grateful for any help readers are able to give 'Bridget's'. I am continually astonished that such good can come out of such evil.

# Material Used

The author is grateful for permission to use the following extracts:

W.H. Auden, "Sext", from *Horae Canonicae*, Faber and Faber Ltd, London 1966

St Augustine, *Confessions*, Sheed & Ward Ltd, London 1987

St Bede, *A History of the English Church And People*, translated by Leo Sherley-Price, Penguin Classics, London 1955 and 1968

Ladislaus Boros, *Pain and Providence*, Burns & Oates Ltd, Search Press, London 1966

T.S. Eliot, "East Coker", from *Four Quartets*, Faber and Faber Ltd., London 1970

Gerard Manley Hopkins, "As Kingfishers catch fire" and "No worst there is none", Oxford University Press, Oxford

Elizabeth Jennings, "Into the Hour" from *Moments of Grace*, Carcanet, Manchester 1979

Harold S. Kushner, *When Bad Things happen to Good People*, Pan Books, London, and Schocken Books Inc., New York 1981

John Masefield, "The Everlasting Mercy" from *Poems by John Masefield*, The Society of Authors as the literary representative of the Estate of John Masefield

H.M. Prescott, *The Man on a Donkey*, Eyre & Spottiswood, London 1953, used by permission of A.P. Watt Limited on behalf of J.W. Prescott and Mrs S.C. Thedinga

Kathleen Raine, "Northumbrian Sequence" from *Collected Poems*, Hamish Hamilton Ltd, London 1956

W.H. Vanstone, *Love's Endeavour, Love's Expense*, Darton, Longman & Todd Ltd, London 1977